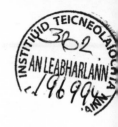

PLEASE DON'T GO

Big John's Journey Back to Life

JOHN HARTSON

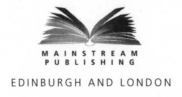

MAINSTREAM
PUBLISHING

EDINBURGH AND LONDON

Copyright © John Hartson 2010
All rights reserved
The moral right of the author has been asserted

First published in Great Britain in 2010 by
MAINSTREAM PUBLISHING COMPANY
(EDINBURGH) LTD
7 Albany Street
Edinburgh EH1 3UG

ISBN 9781845966805 (Hardback edition)
ISBN 9781845966966 (Trade Paperback edition)

All photos courtesy of the author except where stated

A catalogue record for this book is available
from the British Library

Typeset in Caslon and Franklin Gothic

Printed and bound in Great Britain by
CPI Mackays, Chatham ME5 8TD

1 3 5 7 9 10 8 6 4 2

To my wife, Sarah, and my four beautiful children,
Rebeca, Joni, Lina and Stephanie.
You are my life.

Pain is temporary. Quitting lasts forever.
Lance Armstrong

Acknowledgements

I want to say a heartfelt thank you to my parents for being so wonderfully supportive, always.

My family and friends have all helped me more than they will ever know, and my sister Victoria deserves special thanks for allowing me to share the diary she wrote when I was critically ill. Thanks, Vic.

Dr Bertelli, my oncologist, and the staff at the Singleton and Morriston hospitals in Swansea have my greatest respect, and I will be forever grateful to all those who helped me make such a remarkably quick recovery.

Finally, thank you to everyone who is working so hard for the John Hartson Foundation (www.johnhartsonfoundation.com). Here's to the future, and to making a difference.

Contents

Foreword

Anfield, on a March evening, 2003. John Hartson, wearing the green-and-white hoops of Scottish champions, Celtic, receives the ball perhaps 25 yards from the Liverpool goal. This tense UEFA Cup quarter-final tie lies in the balance, with time ticking away. The muscular Welshman digs the ball out of his feet and, with unbelievable power, crashes the ball past a helpless Jerzy Dudek and into the Liverpool net. The goal sends thousands of travelling Celtic fans into delirium and the famous Scottish club into the semi-final of the UEFA Cup. It remains a supreme moment in the history of the club, and the goalscorer instantly catapults himself into Celtic folklore.

Moments like this were what I envisaged when I forced an initially reticent and somewhat reluctant John Hartson away from Coventry, where he enjoyed a wonderful relationship with his manager, Gordon Strachan. John's medical record seemed, on the face of it, none too clever, but I wasn't put off. He hadn't missed too many games in the last few seasons in England, so I took the chance. In fact, it was never a gamble: his goalscoring record with Celtic speaks for itself.

So, I started to get to know the chunky red-haired Welsh international who had looked a world-beater in his very early days at Luton Town. He took a little time to settle in at his new club before blossoming as a natural goalscorer. He and Henrik Larsson formed a magnificent partnership, allowing the wonderfully versatile Chris Sutton to play in a more withdrawn role. As a consequence, with all three in the line-up, goalscoring didn't become a problem for the club.

John's biggest problem was with his weight. He needed to train hard to stay fit, and he wasn't always the best judge of his own fitness. I suppose large breakfasts, early lunches and never-late-for dinners were always going to have an effect on that powerful frame, but, man, he could score goals.

I remember one damp evening at Hampden Park in the semi-final of the League Cup. We had toiled as a team that evening, and John had also done so as a player. I substituted him during the game, but we managed to win through to the final in the end. He was none too pleased with the decision and stormed off down the tunnel. Some moments later, amongst the congratulatory back-slapping and hugging in the dressing-room, Hartson's words ripped through the air. 'Why did you take me off, gaffer?' he asked, with more than a hint of menace in his utterance.

'Sometimes, John, in this game of football you just have to be able to get round the pitch,' I replied sarcastically. 'And by twenty past nine this evening, you just couldn't manage it.' I think now, on reflection, that judging by the physical threat implied in John's question, I might have been wiser to have given that caustic answer from the sanctity of the adjoining coaches' room at Hampden Park.

I was stunned to hear the news that John had cancer. And he was in a critical condition. And still only in his mid-30s. Yet I, more than most, should realise that this desperate disease is no respecter of reputation. It follows no normal path. Some years ago my wife was struck down, and from somewhere deep within herself she found the spirit, willpower and courage to fight back.

John, I felt sure, even in those critical moments, would find similar strength and courage to win his battle. And that is exactly what he has done. I have the utmost regard for that desire to live he has shown. It's great to see him not only alive and well, but also popping up on television doing football punditry. He draws a little smile from my lips when he – very eloquently, I must say – tells us at half-time that if the losing team wishes to improve in the second half, the players will have to work much harder and run off the ball a little more strongly than they had been doing previously. 'John, just tell them how to score a goal; you were great at that,' I shout back at the TV.

As for the future, who knows? His family must just be delighted he is winning his biggest battle. Coaching? Managing? Why not, if John wants it badly enough. But for now, just appreciate the smell of the morning coffee and the sizzle of the frying pan. On second thoughts, John, forget the frying pan and stay healthy.

Good luck in whatever you decide to do.

Martin O'Neill

John's preface

I lay back on the sunlounger and looked at the magnificent view across the Persian Gulf. The water was bright turquoise and the shimmering skyscrapers made me feel as if I was on a film set. Sarah was lying on the beach next to me, and I smiled at her even though she had her eyes shut. She looked beautiful. Sarah always said I was the luckiest person she knew, and right there and then I really felt it. We were in a five-star hotel in Dubai, just the two of us, and it was great to see Sarah relaxing. She's a brilliant mum, but the trouble with brilliant mums is that they never sit still. Lina was just ten months old and completely full on. In fact, life in general was full on, and it was great for Sarah and I to have a complete break together. I sipped a cold beer and thought back over 2009. It was only June, but already we'd been through plenty of twists and turns. At the beginning of the year, I was working for Setanta Sports as a TV pundit and loving it. I'd jumped at the challenge after retiring from football in 2008. People said I took to it like a duck to water. It was true. I love talking about the game and I lapped up the media lifestyle. I can't deny it wasn't a blow when Setanta went bust and I lost my job. I was more than disappointed: I was gutted. But I had other irons in the fire: I was about to complete my football-coaching badges, and I was lining up work with other TV and radio stations. 'Don't worry about a thing,' Sarah smiled when we landed in Dubai.

'Just chill out for five days. Everything can wait; it'll all work out. It always does with you!' It was typical of her. She's a very level-headed, practical Scot, someone good to have on your side. When we met, Sarah was living on the top floor of a Glasgow tenement, and she had her priorities right. She adored her job as an art teacher, and I admired her for being so independent. She had a wide circle of friends and she had lived life to the full, doing an honours degree at the Glasgow School of Art and travelling around Australia with her mates. She really knew how to handle life, and I admired that. I thought back to how gorgeous she had looked at my Celtic tribute dinner at the Glasgow Hilton in March, rubbing shoulders effortlessly with footballers, celebrities and Celtic fans. It was one of the best nights of my life. Gordon Strachan brought the house down with his speech and I was full of pride. 'How can you top this?' I'd thought on the night. I was 34 years old and I'd played top-class professional football for 15 years. I was at an exciting crossroads in my life, but, as ever, I was impatient and wanted to know what would happen next. You couldn't make it up, could you? If someone had told me I'd soon be diagnosed with testicular cancer and almost die, I'd have said, 'You're having a laugh, mate.' I was Big John, the six-foot-two hard nut who went in for killer headers and never flinched. Nothing could bring me down. My body was like a patchwork quilt, I'd had so many cuts from tackles and injuries. I was too tough to be floored by a tiny little lump. Of course, I have learned that nobody is too tough for cancer. It can strike no matter how big and strong or lucky you think you are. I want my story to get that message across. The survival rate for testicular cancer is extremely high when it is diagnosed early. Ignoring a lump can cost you your life. It's that simple. I want to tell how close I came to death in the hope it will save other lives. Sarah is right. I am one of the lucky ones. When I tried to pretend my lump wasn't there, the cancer spread to my lungs and brain. I literally came within seconds of death, but I pulled back from the brink. I don't know how or why I managed to survive, because there were times when I wanted to give up when the pain was just so bad. I thank God I am still here, and I am determined some good will come of my experience and other men won't risk their life through ignorance. Sarah and my younger sister, Victoria, have agreed to help me tell my story, because there were times when I was unconscious or too ill to remember what happened to me in hospital. Victoria wrote a diary. It contains some very personal observations, but I don't mind sharing it if it helps spread awareness. It's the least I can do. I have even wondered if perhaps that is the reason why I got cancer in the first place: because I am in a position to raise public awareness and hopefully help save others going through what I have. Who knows? Who knows why anybody gets cancer? Maybe, for me, this book and the John Hartson Foundation I have created since my illness are my reasons why.

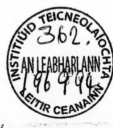

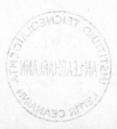

Sarah's preface

John is the luckiest person I've ever met in my life. If anybody else had been diagnosed with cancer and suffered what John has been through, I'd have been terrified they wouldn't survive. But John is one of those people who always comes up smelling of roses. He doesn't just make it through adversity; he comes out the other side with bells on. That's what I love about him, amongst many other things. Before he got ill he was like a walking party, and thankfully that old John is back now. He is loads of fun: his personality fills a room. You feel you can do anything in the world when you're with John, and so many times we did. We ripped it up at parties, jetted off on fabulous holidays and laughed our heads off together whether we were sipping champagne with famous footballers or eating fish and chips at home. Having Lina inevitably changed our lifestyle, but John never changed one bit. He never got bogged down by the demands of parenthood or by the seismic change he went through when he retired from football and became a TV pundit. He has a lovable innocence about him that has never waned. I used to joke that I got on so well with him because he was just like some of the troublesome adolescents I taught. I think people who didn't even know John spotted that youthfulness too and found it endearing. Despite his reputation for being petulant and aggressive on the pitch, fans adored him. As a TV pundit he spoke straight from the heart, winning a new army of fans. When John was in hospital, our house felt half-lit. Our wee daughter Lina kept John's light shining for me, but there was a giant hole in my life without him by my side. As his diagnosis lurched from bad to worse, I never gave up hope. Not having him walk back through the door was unthinkable. The only time I ever really faltered was when he actually stopped breathing and needed an emergency brain operation to save his life. Well, I think I was allowed a little panic attack that day! Now he is back home his personality is filling the empty space again. He rarely complains and doesn't sink into self-pity. He prefers to crack jokes, be the big, indestructible man he always has been and to live life to the full. They are qualities I love and admire – although, of course, it's those same characteristics that made him ignore the lump when he first found it in 2005. Thankfully, John's macho ignorance and embarrassment are the only parts of his personality that have changed in all this. Now he would stand in the middle of Wembley Stadium stark-naked shouting about it if he thought he could stop another man going through what he has (but don't quote me on that!). I know John will be a great ambassador for improving awareness of testicular cancer, and I'm supporting him every step of the way.

Prologue

Maybe I'm going blind. I can't see and I can't keep my eyes open. The pain is flooding in through my eyeballs. I clamp my eyelids shut and curse their frailty. They don't block the pain. If anything the pain intensifies, trapped inside my head like an angry wasp.

I bite my lip to suppress a moan. I cover my eyes with my hands, pressing my palms hard into my eye sockets and digging my fingernails into my scalp.

I feel my warm breath on my wrists. My breathing is slow. I'm keeping very still. I don't want to rattle the pain. I want to sleep. I desperately want to sleep.

I watch the pain as I slowly start to fall asleep. The angry wasp becomes a black shadow in the shape of a large tornado. It is moving very slowly but very purposefully around my head. It twists, corkscrew-like, behind each eyeball in turn, and I grind my teeth as if to form a physical barrier, so the pain can't travel down my throat and torment the rest of my body.

I look deep inside the tornado. It is inky black and its sharp point has found the nape of my neck. It is stabbing me slowly, again and again. My brain is a dense black cloud, hovering perilously above the eye of the storm. I think I am going to pass out.

I am swallowed up by the tornado. I'm in its long dark tunnel. The pain is starting to numb and I can see the tiniest flicker of light at the end. If I can get there I know the pain will go completely. I will be in another place. I will be asleep, fast asleep.

The date is 14 January 1995. I am 19 years old, and I'm walking out of the tunnel and onto a giant pitch. It is so perfectly manicured it looks like a super-sized bowling green. I make out a figure in front of me. It is Ian Wright, wishing me good luck in my Arsenal debut.

Now I am actually standing on the turf at Highbury and a lot of people are watching me. 'Sixty thousand,' I hear a booming voice announce. The voice is drowned out by very loud cheers. It sounds like a million packets of crisps are being scrunched up inside my head.

I feel butterflies in my stomach. A surge of adrenalin shoots round my body and I'm glad of it. It pumps me up, charging me up for the challenge to come.

I see a headline in *The Sun*, 'Graham gets his man', and I snatch at the memory. I am in no pain. I am fit and healthy, brimming with life, buzzing with excitement. I am alive. I am invincible.

I can see flags and arms waving and mouths open wide, but now I can't hear the chants and cheers. All I can hear is the same phrase being repeated time and time again inside my head, in a familiar Welsh accent. 'You've got the world at your feet, boy! You've got the world at your feet!' It's my dad, Cyril's, voice. 'I won't let you down, Dad,' I think. It's a promise I really want to keep. I have to pay him back for everything he has done to help me get this far. I owe him so much.

I allow myself a smile in my dream, and I can see myself smiling. I've got bright-red hair and freckles and a cheeky grin. I am lean and fit and my heart is hammering with pride inside my Arsenal shirt. Its redness feels like it has spilled out from the fire inside my body. I am burning with excitement. My ribs are two radiators, belting out heat. Every pore is red hot. Every eyelash, every fingernail, every whisker.

Now my dream takes me to meet the legendary football manager George Graham in a fancy hotel in north London. I am nervous as hell. My Ford Escort is parked on the gravel outside. It cost my dad £400 and has zebra-striped covers on the seats. The lads at my first club, Luton, take the piss relentlessly, telling me it looks like a Luton minicab.

I will have the last laugh now. I am going to be able to afford a shiny new car. A red Porsche or maybe a silver Bentley? Maybe I'll just get both. I'm not even into cars, but what the hell?

I shake George Graham's hand. I'm in awe of the great man. He signs me for £3,250 a week on a four-year contract. I would have said 'yes' to anything he offered that day.

I'm wearing a tie with Mickey Mouse emblazoned on it, a brown sports jacket that looks a couple of sizes too big and a shirt I borrowed from my landlord. I live in tracksuits or shorts and T-shirts normally. When David Pleat, my Luton boss, told me to 'go home', I had nodded obediently. I thought I was in trouble. I thought I was being shown the door. It wouldn't have surprised me, the way I'd carried on. Instead he said, 'John, put on a shirt and tie and have a shave. You're going to meet George Graham.'

Now the deal is done and I am playing for Arsenal, alongside Ian Wright. He's an England centre-forward, for God's sake. I'm thrilled beyond belief. I can see Dad beaming at me, the same smile he had when he waved me off to play my first football match as a skinny six-year-old lad in Swansea.

My head is throbbing. A week ago I was earning £350 a week playing for Luton. The £2.5-million transfer deal to Arsenal has made me the most expensive teenager in the history of British football. I read the headlines again and again, staring at them in disbelief: 'John Hartson is Britain's most expensive teenager'.

This is the stuff of dreams, but it isn't a dream. This is what happened to me. Signing for Arsenal paved the way for my 15-year career scoring goals for some of Britain's top clubs, as well as earning 51 caps for Wales.

As I lay in my bed at home in Neath for the best part of a week in July 2009, nursing the excruciating headaches that eventually proved to be symptoms of the testicular cancer that nearly killed me, I had many more recollections of my past.

I had time to reflect, time to revel in past successes and time to regret mistakes I have made, of which there are many.

Later, when I was lying in my hospital bed, having escaped death's door, I had more memories still, some triggered by the many cards and letters and messages of support I received from fans and managers and players of all the clubs I played for.

I will tell you about those later. Now, before I tell you what happened to me when the headaches eventually made me pass out for a very long time indeed, I will share some of my earlier memories.

Most involve football, one way or another.

Chapter One

'When I'm big, I'm going be a footballer'

'I've got you a present,' Mam said. 'Go on, open it!'

I ripped the shiny wrapping paper to shreds and jumped for joy when the crinkly plastic packet fell onto the patterns of the living-room carpet.

'Yeeessss!' I shrieked. 'Thanks Mam!' I tore at the plastic with my teeth; it was quicker than looking for the seal. My prize was a bright-yellow football kit. 'Leeds! Look – I've got a Leeds kit!'

Mam beamed. 'I bought you that because it will match your yellow boots,' she said.

'And his red hair,' Dad chimed in.

'Put it on. Let me take a picture!' said Mam.

'Can I wear it when I watch you play next, Dad? Can I?'

I lived for the days when my dad, Cyril, was playing for his team, Afan Lido, in nearby Port Talbot. He was a centre-forward, and at every match I tracked him like an eagle watching its prey. I wanted to be big and strong like my dad. I wanted to be a centre-forward and score lots of goals, just like him. He was awesome.

'Tell me how you scored that second goal, Dad. How did you score from so far away? How did you get the ball off that ginormous defender?'

He loved answering my questions. We'd have talked about football

all day if we could. His eyes lit up when he talked about scoring goals. He had colour in his cheeks, and he just looked so happy.

Mam was happy too. 'What are you boys like?' she'd smile, rolling her eyes in mock sarcasm. 'You're football mad!'

My big brother, James, rolled his eyes too, but he meant it. He had a passing interest in football but didn't share my passion by any stretch.

'Go and read a book, James,' I'd tease. 'Swot!'

He was clever, my big brother. He liked reading, while the only thing I ever wanted to read was the back page of the *Evening Post* to see how Swansea were doing.

My dad was a huge Swansea fan and took me to matches whenever he could. Once I'd got a taste for football kits, he eventually bought me a Swansea strip and a Liverpool one too. Liverpool was my favourite team. I wanted to play for Liverpool one day.

My big sister, Hayley, was clever too. She never missed a trick, or an opportunity to grass her brother up. 'Mam! John's eaten the last Penguin! Mam! John's left his dirty kit all over the bathroom floor!'

Together we were all noisy. We lived in a three-bedroom house on a council estate in Trallwn in Swansea, and sometimes it felt like there were twenty of us in there. Hayley had her music on, I had sport on the telly and Big James was shouting, 'Turn it down! I'm trying to do my homework!'

'What do you do at work?' I asked Dad as we travelled home from one of his football matches. 'Why don't you become a professional footballer?' After playing for Afan Lido he went on to play for Haverford West, who were in the Welsh leagues. The games always felt important. They had proper referees and linesmen and cheering fans. I knew my dad was good, better than most other dads. He got slapped on the back and he scored goals that made his whole team cheer.

Dad was a sign-writer, and he worked for a firm that made and erected 'For Sale' signs. He was proud of his job, and I remember people always said he was a real hard worker. When he shook hands with other men they sometimes winced, he was that big and strong. That made me feel proud of him too.

Mam was a nurse. She had Big James, Hayley and then me all before she was 20 years old. Our baby sister, Victoria, was born when I was seven. She had loads of silky black hair, and I cuddled her in a blanket and asked her if she fancied playing football with me when she was bigger. When she didn't respond, I decided I didn't like her very much. 'Would you like to go in a rabbit hutch or a rabbit hole?' I asked her, and I meant it.

'I'd love to play football for a living, John,' Dad said, exchanging smiles with Mam in the front of his works van, which doubled as our family car. 'But not many people are lucky enough to be able to do that. You have to be really, really good. Maybe you will be lucky, son.'

'Why do you work at night, Mam? Wouldn't you like to sleep at night-time like we do?'

'John, you're a chatterbox today,' Mam said. Both my parents protected me from the adult worries of the world. I know that because I can't remember ever really worrying about anything as a child, except when I was playing football next. There must have been all sorts of issues, bringing up four kids in a small house on a council estate, but I never knew about them if there were.

Mam worked as a nurse at night. She gave us our tea before she went out, and Dad put us kids to bed and often fell asleep in the armchair still wearing his work clothes, he was that tired. I was glad Mam did the tea, because she always made my favourite things, like sausage and mash and egg and chips and beans. I loved my food.

Mam did our breakfast too. Ready Brek, Corn Flakes or toast and marmalade. She was like magic. She reappeared in the kitchen at 7 a.m. every morning, just as if she had never been away.

When Victoria was born I wondered if Mam would have to be even more magical to look after four children, and she was. She didn't take any attention or love away from me or Big James and Hayley. Victoria just sort of slotted in. She slept in a cot in Mam and Dad's room, and my parents seemed to effortlessly spread their love and care around even further.

We were all very different. I shared a bedroom with Big James and I had the top bunk. He'd kick the underneath of my mattress to annoy me, but I was by far the more annoying of the two of us.

'Is that the only kicking you can do?' I teased back. 'Why don't you go and kick a ball instead of reading a book?' Big James enjoyed school, whereas I only went to school for the break times. I kicked a football all the way there, and even when I had to put it in a Spar carrier bag to cross the road I still kicked it relentlessly.

In the classroom I watched the clock. My pulse quickened as the hands turned slowly to 10.15, 12.30 and then 2.30. They were break times and lunch, when I'd tear around the playground kicking my football for all it was worth. I lived for those breaks.

'What are you doing, Big James?' I mocked one day. He was polishing the spokes on his bike. I couldn't believe my eyes. Who polished bike spokes? My bike was covered in mud. You couldn't see the spokes for the dirt. When he'd finished I rode off on his shiny bike laughing my head off, just to annoy him.

'Mam, John nicked my bike! Mam, John's bike is filthy. Mam, why's John so annoying?'

That's how it went. I annoyed the hell out of Hayley too, hogging the TV to watch sport and generally being a boisterous, football-mad little brother.

'Wait till your father gets home!' Mam always warned. 'He'll sort you out!'

We all stopped dead when we heard Dad's van pull up outside our house at Tyn-y-cae Road, Trallwn. The arguments stopped. We froze like statues. The air hung heavy with expectation. Dad's presence did that, even before he opened his van or turned his key in our white front door.

He was a huge man, with big eyes that I imagined saw things other people couldn't see. Maybe he could even see inside my head and know if I was telling lies or thinking bad things?

If Mam was in a good mood she said nothing about our spats, even if we'd run her ragged. If she was at the end of her tether, she still didn't say very much. There was rarely any need. Dad's presence pushed out the chaos and restored order.

When I got older, Mam would boot me out of the house in the evening so Big James could do his homework in peace and quiet. He wanted to be a vet, which kind of baffled me as I thought the only job in the world worth doing was being a professional footballer. I was more than happy to be the scallywag little brother, out on the streets kicking a ball instead of being cooped up in the house.

'Fancy a keepy-up competition?' I said to my best mate, Paul Glover. 'First to 50 – bet I can beat you!'

'No way!' he replied. 'Watch me go. Bet I can top you this time!'

I don't think he ever did, but to this day he's never stopped spurring me on to succeed either. We drove the local shopkeepers mad, kicking footballs up against the walls of Mariano's Fish Bar and the Shahi Indian takeaway.

On Friday nights, Mam and Dad went down the road to the social club. 'Be good,' they smiled, leaving us with a babysitter, a bottle of dandelion and burdock and a six-pack of Salt 'n' Shake crisps.

'What did you do at the club?' I asked the next day.

'I played bingo with my friends, your da played cards and had a couple of pints, and we had a slow dance together at the end of the night and came home at eleven o'clock.'

Mam told me the same thing every time.

Hayley and I went to the local Welsh-speaking school together.

'I'll look out for you,' Hayley told me. I was a tiny, weedy-looking lad, virtually the smallest in the class.

I looked up to Hayley. She was full of fun and good at sport, and I could see she was well liked by the teachers as well as the other kids. She even threw the discus for Wales; how cool was that?

I hated lessons, all lessons. What was the point in science and history when all I wanted to do was kick a football for a living? I remember one parents' evening when I was still a small primary-school child. My teacher looked grave as she beckoned my mum to sit down in a child-sized chair at a tiny table. I didn't care what she was going to say, I just wanted to laugh out loud because Mam looked so funny at that tiny desk.

'John needs to work harder,' my teacher said quite firmly. She took a deep breath and added: 'What if he can't become a professional footballer?'

Mam opened her mouth to reply, but I butted in. 'I will be a professional footballer, Miss. I will. I'm going to play football for my job when I'm big.' There was absolutely no doubt in my mind. I thought my teacher was crazy for doubting me.

I overheard Mam telling Dad how parents' evening had gone.

'Look, Cyril, he's got his heart set on this. He's not interested in school at all. He's getting by, but he's not really trying . . .'

'He's not in trouble, though, is he?' Dad said. 'He's coping with the work. What's wrong with him having a dream? Look, Diana, when I throw the ball to him for a header, he doesn't just nod it back like other kids. He arches his neck, ready to connect with the ball. He was barely out of nappies when he could control the ball with his feet; you know that. It might not be just a dream. John has real talent. He could go all the way.'

I felt like I grew ten feet that night as I hovered on the landing in my *A-Team* pyjamas. Having my dad's seal of approval meant everything to me. I wanted to be as good as him, if not better.

'Fancy joining a team yourself?' Dad asked me one day after I'd watched his team win.

I was six years old. 'Can I, Da?' I asked, open-mouthed. I'd spent the summer holidays practically attached to a football. If I wasn't kicking or heading a ball, I was nursing my favourite football in my arms while I watched the telly.

'I've got you a place with Lonlas Boys' Club,' Dad told me. 'First game this weekend.'

My heart was thumping inside my shirt when we pulled up at the pitch. Everyone called the ground the 'Clinic'. It was at the bottom of the hill in nearby Skewen. It felt like Wembley to me that day.

Much bigger lads than me were warming up. I heard someone say they were under-eights. I squeezed Mam's hand. She was wrapped up in a thick coat and was wearing a bobble hat and chunky scarf.

'Go on, John, good luck,' she smiled, gently guiding me onto the pitch. Her breath left warm white clouds in front of her face. The wind whipped through my shirt and burned the backs of my legs. I wanted to cry.

'Give it your best shot!' Dad shouted with pride. 'That's my boy!'

I walked into the centre of the pitch feeling like a small ice cube lost in a cold sea. The wind whistled around my ears, or was it a real whistle? The other players washed all around me. My knees knocked, and I couldn't see properly through the salty water pooling in my eyes.

Mam and Dad didn't realise. I could see them jumping up and down, bobble hats nodding, hot breath steaming from their smiling mouths. 'Come on, John! Run round and get warm!'

I tried to move my legs, but nothing happened. I was frozen with fear and cold. When a very big man in a black shirt and shorts crouched down beside me and ruffled my hair, tears finally tumbled down my cheeks. 'I want to go home,' I sobbed. 'I'm freezing cold and I want to go home.'

'Go on, run round and get warm!' I heard the shouts from the sideline and I wanted to run, but I just stood rooted to the spot. At half-time I was led off with numb legs and my heart as heavy as a leather ball.

'Never mind,' Mam said with a big smile. 'Let's get you warmed up, love.' She wrapped her arms around me, and the familiar smell of her perfume made me feel better.

Dad said, 'You'll be fine next time.' I looked into my dad's dark-brown eyes and saw something that made my heart instantly feel lighter. Even today I find it hard to describe what I saw, but I will try. It was like looking into a deep well, so deep I couldn't see the bottom. It was full of love and encouragement, inviting me to take as much as I wanted. Willing me, in fact. It was a look I was to see many, many times more as he supported me down the years, often when I didn't deserve his unconditional support.

Dad never pressurised me, at least not in the traditional sense of the word. He wasn't like one of those parents on *Britain's Got Talent*, holding an emotional gun to their kid's head, forcing them to perform, grabbing the reflected glory. No, Dad never did that. But I could see just by looking in his eyes that he wanted the world for me, and he would be disappointed if I didn't make the most of my talent and grab it for myself. I didn't want to disappoint him, I really didn't.

The following week I turned up for Lonlas again, my head ringing with words of encouragement from my dad. 'You can do it, John,' he shouted as I ran onto the pitch. And I did. I played like my life depended on it. I sprinted for the ball like I was doing the 100 m at the Olympics. I controlled the ball as if it was an extension of my boot. I could feel Dad's eyes on the back of my shirt. They were like a power supply, shining an endless beam of energy and enthusiasm into me.

Now when I look back, I can see my dad cheering on the sideline so many times. Just another proud Welsh dad but he was my dad. Him being there always fuelled my hunger for a goal. Whenever I scored, I squealed with delight and looked over to my dad, only to see him bouncing around and shrieking like an excited young boy too. It was a memorable sight, as he was such a giant of a man.

Over the months and years, Lonlas went on to notch up the most amazing victories. On one occasion we won 32–0, and in another game I put twelve goals in the back of the net. We murdered everyone we came up against. I developed a reputation for scoring last-minute winners, and I dreamed of scoring on a big pitch like the ones I saw on telly and the one I saw Swansea perform on when I stood in the stands with my dad.

Playing for Wales, my country, was my ultimate dream. Ian Rush and Mark Hughes were my heroes. I wanted to be like them, and Dad made me believe I could be if I tried my best.

'You have a talent, John,' Dad told me. 'You just need to keep putting in the work, keep improving, keep practising.' That was as close as he came to pressuring me. 'It's down to you, John, at the end of the day; it's down to you, boy. Nobody else can do the work for you.'

I don't know how old I was the first time he said that to me. All I know is that he said the same thing to me over and over again. He never forced me to train or practice when I could have been mucking about with my mates instead. He just consistently pointed out that my future was in my hands – or, rather, at my own feet.

I won the 'Most-Improved Player' award when I was eight. Bonnie Tyler came to Lonlas to present me with my trophy. She smelled absolutely gorgeous, like the beauty counter in JT Morgan in Swansea, and she was in a gold dress that shone as brightly as the cup.

'Well done, John,' she smiled. Her blonde hair dazzled me. She put her arm around me and we posed for photographs. Flash, flash, flash.

I was blinded by the flashbulbs, and my head span like it did when I was on the roundabout in the park, yelling to be pushed faster. If this was what it felt like to be a famous footballer, I wanted it even more.

When winter came, we trained at an indoor barn. The goals were two wooden school benches laid on their sides and the pitch was tiny, but I loved the fast pace of the game in there. I ran myself ragged taking players on. I'd end each session red-faced and saturated in sweat. 'Can't we just have a few minutes more?' I always asked after the final whistle. 'Please?' Some of the other lads couldn't wait to get their drinks and get in the car home. I never wanted it to end, and I wanted to scream and cry if my side didn't win.

I stayed with Lonlas until I was about 12 or 13. By that time I'd built up a reputation as the club's star player and my performances had attracted attention from some of the big clubs. I'd been invited to youth training sessions by the likes of Luton, Leeds and Manchester City. I can't say they were awesome occasions or even that I remember much about them. Dad drove me in his works van and usually it felt like just another game, except it was on a proper, big pitch a long way away. I didn't think it was a big deal, even though my mates back home told me I was dead lucky.

I put my heart and soul into every game, and I'd have smashed though a brick wall if need be to score a goal, but that was what I did in the indoor barn at Lonlas. That's just how I was when I played. I didn't put on a special show for the benefit of the scouts. I simply played every game like my life depended on it. I couldn't understand why a footballer would do anything less.

I remember the first time I heard Bill Shankly's famous quote: 'Some people believe football is a matter of life and death. I am very disappointed with that attitude. I can assure you it is much, much more important than that.' People laughed when they heard it and I wondered why they found it so funny. He was just telling the truth.

'There's a job going in the club,' my mate Karl told me one day. It was the summer holidays. I was 13 years old, and the club he was talking about was the local social club, Barons.

'Doing what?'

'Collecting glasses.'

I kicked my ball against the low wall at the bottom of our road. I was bored.

'How much d'you get paid?'

'£11 a shift. Plus tips.'

My ears pricked up. I kicked my ball all the way to the club and shook hands on my first job. I started that night.

The job itself was a doddle. I enjoyed the chat and the bustle of being in the club, but most of all I liked the feeling I was growing up, earning my own money. Becoming a man. Becoming like my dad.

I was paid on a Friday night. The first time I was handed my pay packet, I felt a rush of blood to my head. It gave me an unexpected buzz. I'd earned nearly 40 quid, and I felt like the big man. Karl and I headed straight to the 24-hour Rileys snooker club, where we played snooker, ate sausage rolls and drank pop until the early hours of the morning.

In between games I had a go on the slot machines. They were the sort of one-armed bandits you put ten pence in and got ten goes. I'd been on them a few times before at fairgrounds and arcades when we'd been on family holidays to caravan parks in Tenby, but this was the first time I'd had plenty of cash in my pocket.

In my mind, my money gave me more chances of winning the big £50 jackpot. I didn't for one moment think of it as a disadvantage, a risk that could make me lose more than ever before. All I saw was the tantalising big-money prize.

Each time I fed another ten-pence piece into the machine, I experienced another buzz. I recognised the buzz, and I welcomed it in. It was the same one I felt when I was about to score a goal. It was like an electrical surge of adrenalin racing through my veins.

My fingers trembled when my last coin clunked into the machine and the red light flashed up: '10 chances'. When I pulled the one-armed bandit, I visualised the three lemons emblazoned with '£50 WIN' flashing before me.

Dreaming of winning. It was a trick I sometimes played on myself when I was about to score. I imagined the ball hitting the net before it actually did, as if my thought waves could give it an extra push. Then I'd roar with victory. 'Goal! Goal! Goal!' All hell would break loose. My brain would throb with delight, and I'd lap up the cheers from the supporters.

The fruits stopped spinning, but now I heard nothing. Silence dropped on me like a wet blanket, snuffing out my excited feelings, numbing my nerves. My last ten pence was gone. I had gambled every last penny of my earnings. There was no victory roar, no fanfare. Just a dim red light flashing: 'No Win . . . No Win . . . No Win . . .' followed by 'Insert Coin Now, Insert Coin Now, Insert Coin . . .'

'I would if I had one!' I shouted, booting the bandit so hard I could hear my wages rattling inside. I wanted to rip the arm off the thing and grab my money back. Not because I felt cheated. Oh no, I didn't feel cheated. I felt that if I could just have a couple more goes, I'd land the big one. That was all I needed. Just a few more goes.

The following week I stayed in Barons long after I got my wages and spent hours on the machines in there. I'd looked forward to winning my losses back and had thought of nothing else all week. Every time I cleared away another glass, I was mentally ticking off the minutes and hours until I could knock off work and hit the machines.

When I walked up to the first one, I had £41.30 in my brown pay envelope. I heard my dad's voice, but thankfully it was only in my head. 'If I catch you near a bandit, boy, I'll whack you round the head,' he had told me after finding out what I'd been up to the week before. Everyone knew my dad and he was well respected on the estate. It wasn't a surprise someone had tipped him off about me playing the fruit machines the week before.

I took a deep breath. He wouldn't ever hit me; I knew that. Dad never once laid a finger on me. I was getting a bit bigger now anyway, just turned 14 and starting to catch up to my dad's height. I wasn't afraid of anyone. I was a big man now, earning my own money. I was entitled to do what I liked.

I lost all my earnings again. It felt like a physical blow to my stomach when I heard my last ten pence land in the bowels of the bandit. By the Tuesday I was desperate to play again, and when Mam wasn't looking

I slipped my hand into her handbag and felt around for her purse. I opened it inside the bag and tightened my palm around a fifty-pence piece.

It was enough to allow me a few more games on the bandits. I didn't think of it as theft. It wasn't stealing, was it? It was only fifty pence, and besides, playing the bandits was something I just had to do. Not playing the machines was not an option. My nerves were snapping around my body like elastic bands. My fingers were itching to pull the machines. It was a physical need I had to satisfy. Mam wouldn't miss it, would she?

I had my first cigarette around this time too. My clothes would reek of smoke whenever I worked in the club, so I didn't think anyone would notice if I actually smoked a cigarette myself.

'Let me smell your breath,' Dad demanded as soon as he opened the front door that night. 'Have you been smoking?'

I nodded, chin scraping my chest. 'What are you doing, son, you're not one of them,' he said. His words chilled me. They echoed round my head. 'You're not one of them.' I felt truly ashamed. I thought of the hours I'd put in at football training, pushing my body so hard my chest hurt. I thought of the trials I was going to.

Since the age of 13, I'd spent my school holidays going for trials up and down the country. My future depended on my body. I didn't have much hope of getting O levels or CSEs, as I put in the bare minimum of effort of school. But I had feet that could kick a ball into the middle of next week and a skull so strong I'd have headed a shot put if anyone had asked me to. My lungs were my power supply, firing me up like a couple of generators.

Filling them with smoke suddenly seemed so stupid. 'I'm sorry, Dad, I won't do it again.' I meant it.

As I spoke the words I knew I was saying the right thing, but sometimes just knowing the difference between right and wrong isn't enough. There was a little red devil lurking inside me. He was the one that made me bunk off school sometimes, knock on people's doors and run away and pelt balls at the windows of Mariano's Fish Bar. That devil grew with me. He became bigger and more aggressive when I started playing the fruit machines, and I found him harder to ignore.

At 15, he grew again and started messing with my head.

'I don't want to play football any more,' I told my dad one day. To this day I don't know why I was rebelling and pressing the self-destruct button, but I couldn't help it. Perhaps I was afraid of failure? I will never know, but thankfully my dad continued to offer me the bottomless pit of support he had done since my first shambles of a performance on a pitch as a six year old.

'Are you mad?' he asked. 'You are being watched constantly by the English league clubs now, boy. They can see your potential, John. With the right discipline and good coaching, you could make the big time. You could achieve your dream. Imagine me and your mam coming to watch you play for Wales? Imagine that? You're no ordinary player, John. Don't waste your talent.'

I thought about my mates. They were starting apprenticeships, getting their hands dirty doing jobs I never wanted to do, fitting double glazing and plastering walls.

Big James had passed his exams with excellent grades and decided on a career as a policeman.

But I didn't have a hope in hell of leaving school with any qualifications that would land me a decent job. I didn't want an ordinary job. I wanted to play football for a living.

It took me three months to come to my senses and start training again. In the end, it wasn't the fear of what I would do with myself if I didn't become a professional footballer that got me going again, it was purely the love of football. I missed it. I missed the thud of my boot on the ball, the heart-pumping training sessions and, above all, the sheer pleasure of scoring a goal. I threw myself back into training and took up every offer of a trial that came my way. This was my future, but I had to make it happen. As usual, Dad was right.

A letter arrived for me one Thursday. I knew it was Thursday as that was the day when Mam would spend about £70 doing the weekly shop and the house would be full of pop, chocolate biscuits and crisps. Every week Mam would shout, 'When it's gone, it's gone – I'm not buying any more until next Thursday!' and we'd all say 'OK, Mam, OK,' ignore her and tuck in. There were rarely any goodies left by the weekend.

On this particular Thursday, I found a letter on the mat as I helped Mam carry in the shopping. It was addressed to me, and it had a Luton FC emblem stamped across it. I don't think I'd ever had an official letter addressed to me before. It felt important.

I thought back to when I was ten years old. That was the first time I was invited to Luton, on the back of my winning performances at Lonlas. The memory of that day was locked in the back of my mind, but I'd never really given it a second thought until I held this letter in my hand.

Suddenly I had a vivid recollection of how David Pleat asked me to sit beside him in a fancy office, and asked me what I wanted to eat later. I asked for beans on toast, and that is what I got. It seemed quite normal at the time, but I guess it was anything but. I guess that is why my dad kept on at me. Things like that didn't happen to most ten-year-old boys.

I'd already played a few matches for Luton's youth team, but this letter changed my life. It offered me a place on the Luton Youth Training Scheme from the age of 16, for the sum of £26 a week. They were taking me on, offering me a real start. I was actually going to be paid to play football.

'Mam – read this!' I shouted. 'I'm joining Luton!'

Mam cried. She cries at everything. She gave me a hug and told me she would miss me like mad, but she wished me luck. She said the same thing as she waved me goodbye with tears splashing down her cheeks after she and Dad had driven me to Luton in his white van.

I remember sitting in my bedroom in my digs and wondering what to do next. Mam and Dad weren't here any more. I had one record in my bag, a Meat Loaf album, and I took it out and played my favourite track, 'Two Out of Three Ain't Bad', over and over again. The lyrics made me think of the meeting I'd attended earlier at Luton, and I laughed.

There had been eighteen of us YTS lads assembled, and we were told in no uncertain terms that Luton expected an awful lot from us over the next two years, especially in terms of physical work. I thought of scoring goals. Two out of three wouldn't be good enough. I was being paid for my football now, trained by a proper club. Playing football for a living, just as I wanted to. I needed to score three out of three now. I was beyond excited, and I felt pumped up for the challenge.

Chapter Two

Living the dream

My fingers trembled as I pressed the buttons. 'Select amount you wish to withdraw.' I pressed on £50 and snatched the five crisp tenners almost before the machine had finished spitting them out.

I swallowed hard and hurried to the arcade. 'Nobody will ever know,' I chanted in my head. 'Nobody will ever know.' I had beads of sweat on my forehead and was flushed with colour as I fed the first note into the change machine and filled my pockets with coins.

I felt good. I was still trembling, but with excitement now instead of nerves.

The clatter of the bandit flicking the fruits around excited me more each time. My heart clattered too, pumping the blood excitedly around my body and making me feel almost dizzy with the thrill of it. The feeling lasted for hours, until the last penny had disappeared down the throat of the fruit machine. I scrabbled in my pockets, hoping to find just one more ten pence, but I was cleaned out.

I walked back to my digs feeling a bit sick and guilty, just as I used to when I'd scoffed the last of the chocolate biscuits and lied about it to Mam. Joan and Steve Goodfellow had kindly taken me in as a lodger. Their son Scott was also in the Luton youth team.

'I've done sausage and mash tonight, John,' Joan smiled brightly. 'Tuck in now. You lads need to keep your strength up!'

My stomach was empty and I wanted to eat, but the food stuck in my throat. I looked at Scott and thought of the cash card in the back pocket of my jeans. It had his name stamped across the bottom, not mine. And somehow I had to put the card back on his bedside table and hope he didn't miss it, or the cash I had withdrawn from his account.

Suddenly the card felt like a flashing light, glowing brightly, yelling out to all Goodfellows, 'Look at me! The lad you've given a home to and looked after like a son has stolen from you! He can't help himself! He is addicted to fruit machines. How sad is that!'

I felt embarrassed and pathetic and couldn't look any of them in the eye. When the truth eventually surfaced a week or so later, the embarrassment turned to deep shame and guilt that gave me a horrible pain in my chest for a very long time.

Dad didn't have to say much. He looked physically crushed as he sat in his favourite brown armchair in our front room at Tyn-y-cae Road.

'Let me get this right. You have thrown away your dream at the age of 16 for a cheap thrill on the bandits?'

I thought of all the hours he had stood on rain-soaked touchlines supporting me, all the miles he had driven me in his van even when he was dog-tired after working all week, and all the words of encouragement he had given me since I was a small boy.

Mam cried. I wanted to crawl under the floorboards and never come out.

Waking up was a daily punishment. As soon as I opened my eyes and saw my old blue-striped duvet cover on my bunk bed, I remembered what had happened.

I relived the shame over and over again, and I dreaded the news from Luton. I'd been sent home in disgrace. I was a petty thief and a gambler, and I was just 16. Would David Pleat give me a second chance? I was terrified, and the waiting seemed to go on for ever.

'You're a lucky boy,' Dad told me one morning without smiling. 'Now pack your bags; I'm taking you back to Luton. You will get no more chances. I told you, you make your own luck in this world. Don't you dare waste your talent again. Work hard. Do your best. You've got the world at your feet, do you hear me, boy? You've got the world at your feet.' I nodded and packed in silence, my heart doing somersaults with relief and excitement.

Dad's words were to ring in my ears many more times throughout my career, and I am ashamed I didn't always listen to them.

But at 16 I did listen to every word he said. The shock of nearly losing my chance of becoming a professional footballer before I'd even started spurred me on, and the pain I felt when I thought of letting him and my mam down fuelled my ambition. I kept my head down, and for my meagre £26 wage – less than I earned collecting glasses in the club at home – I trained and played like an absolute demon.

Lying in bed alone at night in my digs at the Goodfellows' – yes, incredibly, they took me back in – I'd dream about scoring goals for the first team. I wanted to prove I could hack it, prove to my dad I was sorry and that I was worth sticking by. I was almost angry with determination every time I kicked a ball, and I developed an aggressive edge that stayed with me throughout my career. I had fire in my belly, and I was going to light up every pitch I played on.

I got my chance to prove myself on 28 August 1993. I was 18 years old when I made my debut for Luton against Nottingham Forest.

My stomach lurched when I ran out onto the pitch. They had Stuart Pearce, Vance Warner, Steve Chettle and Des Lyttle in the back four. They were men. I felt like a small boy by comparison, despite my fully grown aggression and the fact I had shot up to at least six feet by then.

It was blazing hot. My legs felt on fire and my head was burning. I ran in for a cross and connected with the ball, directing a header into the back of the net. In that moment, my whole world made sense. Dad's words of warning and encouragement. The physical effort I put into training. Hauling myself around a frozen pitch in the deep of winter until my lungs almost cracked. Moving away from home, so far away from my friends and family.

Now I knew why. For the first time, I could actually feel my dream coming true. I was living it right there and then. I could smell it and touch it and hear it. The sickly smell of wet grass and fresh mud, the hot drops of sweat making tracks down my tingling spine and the eruption in the crowd bouncing around my eardrums: everything was supercharged. Nothing had ever felt so good as that moment. I was drenched and dizzy with satisfaction, but I craved more. Scoring goals was the best thing in the world, and I wanted the next one even more than the last.

'How d'you feel?' Dad asked me after the match.

'Magic,' I said. 'I never want this to stop.' His lips stretched into a broad smile that seemed to smooth away every line from his face.

I went on to make forty-two appearances for Luton, scoring six league goals and one in the FA Cup. Each one was magical.

Unfortunately, I still got magical kicks from fruit machines too.

Winning a couple of quid gave me similar feelings to scoring a goal. 'I never want this to stop,' I thought as I fed in the last of my wages week after week. Deep down I knew what I was doing was wrong and I felt ashamed of being addicted to fruit machines, but I just couldn't stop.

It was a cold, wet Wednesday in October 1993. I was penniless, even though by now I earned £350 a week, much more than all of my mates back in Wales. I thought about home. I thought about kicking a ball down my street with Paul Glover and sitting round the kitchen table eating roast chicken with Big James and Hayley and Victoria and Mam and Dad. The image gave me a warm, comfortable feeling inside, like a little valve had been switched and just the right amount of pressure had escaped from my body.

'Hartson, can I have a word?' It was David Pleat.

'Yes, boss.' The gas had been lit again and my pulse quickened. I was working hard. The cash-card incident was behind me. What now? I clenched my stomach muscles and pulled myself up tall. I had to be strong, even though in that moment I didn't feel it. I just wanted to go home and escape all the pressure I was under and the relentless need to prove myself.

'You've been called up to play for Wales. First match an under-21 international against Cyprus.'

His words bounced around my head switching on lights like a marble in a pinball machine.

'Thanks for telling me. That's great news. Thank you.' I wasn't sure

I had managed to string a sentence together. I wanted to jump up so high I could punch the ceiling, but I bit my lip and kept my cool. 'Thank you,' I smiled. I could feel a surge of pressure in my belly. 'Bring it on!' I thought. 'Bring it on!'

Now, I'm lying in bed at home in July 2009, returning to these memories, dreaming about my dreams and how they played out in real life. The headaches interrupt them, but they don't shut them out, not just yet.

I remember a series of snapshots, like I'm flicking though a photo album in my mind. The images I recall evoke powerful emotions.

I see my serious expression as I stand on the pitch before the Wales v. Cyprus match. The Welsh national anthem brings a lump to my throat. I've looked forward to singing this as much as I've looked forward to the match. I think of my mam and dad in the crowd; I want to make them proud. My grandmother, Annie, who we all called Mamgu – Welsh for 'Nan' – has wished me luck. We all love Mamgu to bits, and I desperately want to tell her afterwards, 'I helped Wales win!'

I can smell the newness of the red number-nine shirt on my back. It is sticking to me already. I can feel moisture in every crease in my skin and in every root of my hair. I have floppy ginger hair and a goatee, and my thighs are like a couple of gnarled tree trunks, I've trained so hard.

My mind explodes. The ball is in the back of the net. Not once, but twice. I feel I have grown on the pitch. I am floating, and my head is skimming the clouds. Mam is crying and kissing me and Dad doesn't need to say a word. He smiles at me and he is oozing pride from every pore, from the well that runs deep inside him.

I turn the photo album in my mind. I'm deep in dreamland, but my dreams are real memories, not make-believe.

I'm at Arsenal. David Pleat has fixed up my deal with George Graham, and I am the most expensive teenage footballer in Britain. I'm delighted and nervous all at once. I have a cocktail of feelings mixing and shaking inside me, making every cell in my body bubble and fizz.

Now I'm scoring my first goal for Arsenal. It's a winning goal against

Coventry. All my nerves are exploding. I'm jumping and being jumped on. My heart is thumping in my chest.

I'm a giant when I leave the ground. I'm stopping at the late-night garage to buy the first editions of the Sunday papers. I'm there on the back page, celebrating with my arms in the air after scoring for Arsenal. I look at myself in disbelief. I am 19 years old. I am living my dream.

That memory ends, and the euphoria slips down my throat. I gulp. My stomach is tense and knotted. I see Bruce Rioch's face. He has replaced Stewart Houston as manager at the end of my first season. I am gutted. I am nervous. I don't know this man, and he doesn't know me. He leaves me out of the team. I feel bullied. I sit on the bench, and as I watch the other players run onto the pitch, week in, week out, I see a pale ghost of myself running back down the tunnel. Is this the end of the dream? It can't be over so soon.

I see Arsène Wenger walking towards me. He is a curious Frenchman I know nothing about. He is my manager now. He gives me cereal and supplements, carrots and grilled fish when I want to eat steak and chips, but I don't argue. He has style. He makes me stretch after training. I do as I'm told. I'm earning £4,000 a week and trying my very best, but still I feel frustrated.

In twenty-six appearances I score just four goals. I'm hungry as hell. I want more headlines. I want to be King of Highbury. Every match feels like a trial, as well as a battle. I pick up ten yellow cards.

On 1 January 1997 I feel like a raging bull when I run out onto the pitch against Middlesbrough. The ref makes a bad decision and the red mist comes down. 'Shithouse,' I snarl. He hears. I meant him to hear. He sends me off. I now have eight bookings against me in my last eleven games.

In my mind, the ref doesn't just send me off the pitch at Highbury, he sends me away from Arsenal. That's how it felt, and that's how it played out.

I am sold for £3.3 million to West Ham. The money is mind-boggling. Suddenly I feel worth my weight in gold.

I celebrate with a bet. Forget the fruit machines. I can gamble big money now. I am gambling heavily. I can't resist the thrill I get from gambling. Will I pull off a huge win? I really want to win big money.

Am I mad? No. I am successful. I'm earning £6,000 a week working out my contract at Arsenal. I can afford to pay the bills and gamble big money. What's wrong with that?

I don't go into the bookie's now. People might recognise me. I set up telephone accounts and keep my gambling secret from everyone.

I am £30k down on one account. I have never been in debt because of my gambling, and I don't intend to stay in debt on this account. I pick a foreign football match to gamble on, to wipe the slate clean.

'Put me £2k on the draw at 9/4, £2k on 0–0 at 7/1 and £2k on no score at 9/2 . . .

'And I want £2k on half-time and full-time scores being the same at 6/1.'

I am in the lounge at Brookmans Park. I am married to my first wife now. This is my five-bedroom mansion set in an acre of parkland in Hertfordshire. It has a full-sized football pitch and paddocks out the back. Nobody can see me. The electric gates are locked. I am all alone. I can hear myself breathing as I watch every frame of the match.

I grip the remote control, almost snapping it in two when the ball hits the woodwork.

When a penalty is missed in the closing minutes, I allow myself a low cheer. I swig a beer nervously. Sixty seconds to go. If it stays 0–0, I will clear £60k. I will clear my debt.

'And on the final whistle it's a disappointing nil–nil draw . . .' I laugh at the commentator.

I am dancing round the living room on my own. 'Disappointing to everyone but me!' I am dialling the bookie's, claiming my win. And I am already planning my next bet.

I am lying to people now. I have a code when I phone the bookies. When I say £100, the bookie knows I mean £1,000. If I say £2,000, I really mean £20k. If anyone is listening, it doesn't sound too bad. If I lose £20k one day, nobody knows.

There is still petrol in the Bentley and the Porsche and the Jeep and the Audi, and plenty of food in the fridge. My house is safe, and I have savings and investments.

I feel a surge of disappointment whenever I lose, but I know it will quickly become a craving to stake more, increase the odds, win more back than I have lost. I haven't lost. If I am down today, there is always tomorrow.

'John, I'm home!' The familiar Scottish voice startles me but comforts me all at the same time. I flick my eyelids open for a moment. Light streams into my eyes and fuels my headache. I want to shut my eyes, but I want to see where I am. I see a photo of Sarah and Lina propped up on the dressing-table. Thank God I'm at home, and Sarah is here. I am in my bed at home in Neath in July 2009, and the gambling is a distant memory. Thank God.

'John, shall I make us a cup of tea before I go to the nursery for Lina . . . ? How are you feeling? Any better?'

'Thanks, babe.' The clink of the mug on the glass coaster on the bedside table sends a shockwave through my head. 'I'm fine thanks, Sarah. I'll drink that and have another little sleep. Head's still not great. You carry on; I'll be fine after a bit more sleep. See you later. You OK?'

I close my eyes and invite sleep back in. I crave it. It's like a fleecy blanket I can rest my brain in for a little while to cushion the pain.

I let my mind wander back down the years, and as sleep draws closer I pick out a good memory, something to try to make me feel better.

I remember being at Ascot on a crisp, bright day. I am in my early 20s and I have £10k cash in my pocket. I wouldn't have gone to the races with anything less. I can see my horse nosing ahead, the hot air from his nostrils warming the tail of the horse in front. 'Go on, go on.'

He inches forward. I am on my feet. I shout his name. It has something to do with hearts. The odds were pretty good, of course, but that was what made me pick this horse: because his name sounded vaguely like mine. That's as technical as I got.

I'm screaming so hard my lungs are blown up like balloons. His nose wins it and I am bouncing in the air, punching huge fists into the sky, waving my winning ticket.

I float out of Ascot in a bubble of champagne. I have £67k in a Sainsbury's carrier bag. I put it in the boot of my Audi and calmly place my golf clubs on top to hide it.

I am in control. I am controlling my excitement. I crave more and more, and I am allowing myself more and more. And why shouldn't I? I sell the Bentley for £85k. I've owned it for all of six months and it cost me £115k. I've lost £30k. It's just a week's wages or a few good wins on the horses. So what?

I blink. I am back in the present again, and a wave of pain cascades from the back of my eyes to the nape of my neck.

I am lying in bed, paralysed with pain, and I'm 34 years old. This fact takes a moment to filter through to my brain. I have a mortgage on the house. I have mortgages on other houses too. I have three children to provide for, and another on the way. What if these headaches are something really bad? What if I can't pay my mortgage? What if I can't feed my children?

I picture little Lina giggling. I think of my mam and dad, always providing for me and my brother and sisters. We always had clean clothes and plenty to eat. It didn't matter that we lived on a council estate. Mam and Dad gave us security and love and protected us from harm and worry. I had to do the same for Lina and the new baby. I had to do the same for Bec and Joni, my children from my first marriage. What if I couldn't?

My head is throbbing and a deep fear grips at my insides. I feel icy cold. I pull the duvet over my head slowly, so as not to rattle the headache.

As the hours and, eventually, the days slip by, I carry on my journey of memories. Having left Arsenal, I am scoring goals regularly for West Ham. We nearly get a European place and I nearly get the Premiership Golden Boot award with my tally of 24 goals in 1997–98. Nearly.

Nearly isn't good enough. I want to be a hero, but I'm not.

I'm locked up in a cell in Epping Police Station. I open my eyes slowly. My head is banging. I see my Uncle Keith and close my eyes again. Tell me this isn't happening. I remember. We had one too many last night and Uncle Keith decided to help himself to the bar at the Epping Forest Country Club.

'West Ham Star in Late Night Row'. This dream is turning into a nightmare. I see another headline. I make it out in my mind. I hope it's a good one. It's not. A barman is accusing me, wrongly, of headbutting him in a bar in Southgate. I remember clearly what happened. We had a tiff when he cleared away my drink before I'd finished.

I'm getting irritated. The *News of the World* is phoning me. 'We hear you have gambling debts of £130,000, John.'

I am at Gamblers Anonymous in a dimly lit room in St Albans. 'Hello, my name is John Hartson. I am a footballer and I am addicted to gambling. I don't really want to stop, but I am upsetting people I love.'

'You have to want to stop for yourself too, John.'

A dozen pairs of eyes watch me, waiting for me to say it. Waiting for me to say that I, John Hartson, want to stop gambling, but I can't. I look at the floor. I am sitting on a metal chair in small grey room. It is depressing. I feel like a fool. I want to get out quick.

'OK. I will try. I really will try.' I have no real intention of trying, because I don't think I have a real problem. I am lucky, because I can afford my addiction.

Next, three officers are grabbing me. They are wearing riot gear. I feel the cold metal of the handcuffs as my arms are clamped behind my back and I'm thrown in the back of a van.

I am in a cold, dark police cell. I am on my own. I relive the events of the evening. There are five of us out on the town in Swansea. One of my old mates takes down an ornamental hanging basket and chucks it at me. I kick it. Everyone laughs and shouts, 'Goal: 1–0, Hartson.' It is caught on CCTV. I fast-forward my brain. I am in court. I am charged with criminal damage and fined £60. I am the Wales centre-forward, and I am made an example of. I am an idiot.

I see red. My blood is up. I am angry now. I am training at Chadwell Heath. Eyal Berkovic is training with me. I admire this man. He is unselfish up front. He makes lots of goals for me at West Ham.

We have been beaten 2–0 by Northampton in our last League Cup game. It is September 1998 and I am 23 years old.

'What went wrong?' demands Harry Redknapp. He is fuming. He wants answers and demands one from each of us. I want to give him what he wants. I respect Harry and we are friends. He likes a bet, like me, and we go to the dogs together. I speak from my heart. I am trying to help Harry to help us win. 'I wouldn't play Eyal away from home,' I say.

It infuriates Eyal. His dark eyes blaze like hot coals. He accuses me of not running for the ball away from home, or any other time. He swears. He is mad as hell.

We are on the training field now. I can see our orange bibs and the steam rising from our hot heads in the cold air. John Moncur rolls the ball in my direction and Eyal intercepts it. I charge in from behind and take his legs away. He rolls on the floor, squealing in pain. I am instantly sorry, and I try to help him up.

I offer my hand and I pull him off the ground, but he lashes out unexpectedly, punching me in the stomach. I catch my breath in shock. It hurts. Suddenly I have no control over my legs. I am absolutely blazing with fury. My left boot shoots out and cracks Eyal under the jaw. I kick him hard, like I'm trying to score a goal with his head. That's what he told me it felt like afterwards.

Eyal is squirming in agony now. I know this is wrong, very wrong. In my dream, I feel myself squirm in my bed as I recall this memory. I am deeply ashamed, as ashamed today as if it has just happened. I will never, ever get over that shame. I wish I could turn back the clock and erase the memory. I can't, and I will always deeply regret it.

Another memory. I am heading for Wimbledon with my spirits low. My reputation is in tatters. I have picked up two red cards and ten yellows in my two years with the Hammers. I have been locked up twice and my gambling habit has been exposed in the press. When footage of me kicking Eyal in the head is played on *News at Ten* the newsreader warns parents that the clip is so disturbing they may want to send their children out of the room.

Wimbledon pays £7.5 million for me. I sigh deeply in my bed, in my dream. Is it regret or relief? Relief, I think. Things can't be that bad. I am offered more than £20,000 a week. That's good, but it's not about the money. I am not in this to fill up a bank-book. I am in this to fulfil my childhood ambition and make my family proud. Being paid that amount of money pleases me greatly because it means I am highly thought of as a player. That's what really matters to me. That, and being able to afford the odd flutter without compromising my lifestyle.

I want to shine and I want to put the misdemeanours of West Ham behind me. In my dream I see doors slamming in my face, and I remember it doesn't work out as I had hoped. I don't want to think about it. I am out of the top league and in and out of a relegated team. I slam the door shut. I don't want to think about it any more.

I'm losing heart. I am not enjoying my football. I am looking for something else to give me the buzz.

I buy a hospitality box at Selhurst Park for £30k. I'm not holding down a regular place on the team. I want to have some fun. When I know I am not playing, I invite my mates over. We drink champagne. I'm having a lot of fun now. It's not my fault I'm not playing, is it? The club is going though major upheavals. I remember them vividly and I flick through them in my mind.

Joe Kinnear, the Wimbledon manager, suffers a heart attack and has to leave the club just months after I sign. I miss him greatly.

Sam Hammam sells the club to a Norwegian consortium that brings in new manager Egil Olsen. I don't rate him. I burn with embarrassment when I remember how I slagged him off in a post-match interview with Sky.

We had just lost 3–0 to Bradford at the end of the 1999–2000 season. I'd been sent off, and when the Sky reporter asked me the fateful question, 'What is wrong with the team?', I let rip, tearing into Egil's management style. If someone asks me an honest question, it's in my blood to give an honest answer. I shut my eyes. Not long after that, Wimbledon decide to sell me.

Now I can see a black storm on the horizon. It is raging, building up speed, wreaking havoc. I am in the eye of the storm, being thrown about. I have no control. My head bangs harder just thinking about it.

A thunderbolt strikes and I am trapped in a dark tunnel. I can't get out.

The bolt startles me, and I look around, sweating. I am relieved to see I am still in my own bed, back in the present day. I shudder when I realise what the tunnel was in my memory. It was a CAT-scan tunnel.

I roll on my side, curled up in a ball like a little boy. I never want to have a CAT scan again. I want my head to stop hurting. I never want to go to a hospital ever again.

It is quiet in my room and the house is empty. I wish Sarah were here. I wish I could get up and go for a round of golf, but I can't move. I'm afraid if I do anything, whatever is storming round my head will get even angrier, and maybe even explode. I am forced to lie still and close my eyes. I really hate being alone and I really hate the dark. I can't stop myself panicking about going to hospital, reliving the past horrors of my failed medicals.

It was 2000 when Wimbledon decided to sell me. Am I dreaming about this, having a nightmare about it or just reliving it though these torturous headaches? I'm not sure. My mind is all over the place.

I snatch at some good memories that trickle through. I am being voted Scottish Professional Footballers' Association Players' Player of the Year, and I win the coveted Scottish Football Writers' Association Player of the Year. I am scoring my 100th goal for Celtic against Falkirk, and I am scoring against Hearts on 5 April 2006, my 31st birthday. I will never forget those landmarks. They remind me that I made it through and I want them to stay and comfort me, but I can't stop my mind returning to the horrors of those medicals. I hate scans and hospitals, I really do.

The first club to approach Wimbledon was Tottenham, managed by my old Arsenal boss George Graham. They offered me £25,000 a week over four years.

I had a routine medical with scans on my knees and hips. I can't remember all the details; I just remember the hammer blow. It came from David Pleat, my old Luton boss, by then a director at Spurs.

'I'm sorry, John, the doctors feel your medical problem, your knee, *is* a problem.'

The words both surprised and baffled me. I didn't know I had a medical problem. I was training as usual; nothing was hurting me. I didn't believe I had a medical problem. I shrugged and felt a shiver of disappointment. 'It wasn't meant to be.' That's what I told myself. The headlines hurt more. 'Hartson Fails Medical.' Ouch.

That night I looked at my daughter Rebeca, sleeping calmly in her pretty pink bed, surrounded by fluffy bunnies and teddy bears. She was just a baby, and I needed to provide for her. What if I really did have a problem? What if my career was over?

'Don't be stupid.' I gave myself a talking-to. 'Tottenham just wasn't meant to be, John. You're in your prime; you know that. You're twenty-five years old, lean and fit and solid. The scan was a blip, an inexplicable blip, that's all.'

I kissed Bec goodnight and told myself to look forward, not back. I mentally buckled myself in. I was on a journey and I didn't have a clue where I was going to end up, though I sensed it wasn't going to run smoothly. Nothing ever does in football.

Lying in bed now, I remember that talking-to I gave myself, and I attempt to repeat the conversation in my head. The headaches are crashing around. I see Lina's face, and she looks the same age as Bec in my memory. 'Just a blip, an inexplicable blip. It will all come good. It always does. You're lucky, John, that's what everybody says. That's what Sarah always says.'

The words are hanging heavy in the warm summer air as I chivvy my memory along, encouraging my mind to move forward from the Tottenham disappointment. I can't cope with any extra pain right now; I want to escape my pain. I close my eyes and snatch at sleep. It's irritating. My brain won't switch off from the memories or the pain. I don't know what is causing my headaches, and I don't know what is worse: the hammering pain or the crushing memories.

I am feeling very low, and trying to be positive is a struggle. I'm not patient. I want results and I want them now. I want to know what is happening to me.

The next day, Charlton Athletic offered £5.5 million, depending on the results of yet another medical. It was half a million less than Spurs but still big money, by far enough to keep me in the game.

'Just a blip, that scan.'

The words are mocking me now. I know by now they are not true. This scan business was turning into much more than a minor blip in my career. It was destroying it.

I remember sitting inside MRI machines, being scanned all over my body for hour after hour. It is mind-numbingly boring. I never wanted to have to do that again.

'Sorry, John.' I can hear Alan Curbishley's voice now, the manager at Charlton. 'Can't do it. I'm afraid the transfer is off. It's the knee.'

I swallowed hard. My heart contracted in my chest. This was harder to stomach. What if I really did have a problem? What if this 'weakness' two scans had identified was going to finish my career at the age of twenty-five?

Two months passed. I was scoring goals for Wimbledon, making a mockery of the scan results. You know when something is wrong with you, don't you?

Like now, lying in bed, rigid with pain. There was something wrong with me. My headaches were nailing my head to the pillow, making it impossible for me to move, let alone get up.

But the knee? No, it wasn't real. It was a phantom problem.

I shut my eyes and winced. Two sentences collided painfully behind my eye sockets. 'Rangers want to pay six million quid for you and they want you at Ibrox for a medical immediately.' It was Mark Hughes' voice, manager of Wales, excusing me from a Wales v. Belarus match so I could fly up to Glasgow and do the deal of a lifetime. Rangers laid on a private jet, they were so keen to get me up there. It all happened so fast.

'I'm sorry. I can't do it.' That is Dick Advocaat's voice, manager of Rangers. I can still hear his words clearly. 'I'm sorry. I can't do it.' I was a Wales international, but I had failed another medical.

The nails in my head took another pounding. My head hurt so much. I felt sick. I wanted to throw up. And then a third voice, a soothing Welsh voice, rubbed away some of the pain. 'Don't worry, son, you'll be back and you'll be back stronger after this.' My dad, of course. He was in the plane with me, flying home, telling me everything would turn out well in the end.

I felt sorry for myself, then and now. It wasn't fair. Why did I have to go through this? Why was I being punished like this?

Coventry came next. The word made my heart sink. They were second from bottom in the Premiership. Gordon Strachan was managing them, helping them fight for survival. He wanted my help. I was trying to survive too, but I failed. I failed my fourth medical. My fourth transfer attempt was in tatters. It must have been some sort of a record, but certainly not one I wanted to hold. My spirits sank. The pep talks I had given myself couldn't possibly wash any more. This was no blip. I was washed-up.

'Gordon, I've got my beautiful daughter Rebeca at home who needs me. I just want to go home and hold her, and then I want to shut the door and bury my head in a blanket. I'm sick and tired of all this.'

Blackness descended. Three long days and nights of the blackest mood. Everywhere I looked was black, and even inside my head it was coal-black. My skull was a dark cave, and I couldn't imagine light shining in ever again.

It was Gordon's voice down the phone that finally broke through, chipping away at the concrete that had set hard and cold around my brain.

Wimbledon had agreed to sell me for £4.5 million to Coventry. I would be paid £20,000 a week on a four-year contract despite failing the medical. Very slowly, Gordon's words let light into my world again.

I blinked in their brightness, weighing up the pros and cons.

It was certainly a way out of Wimbledon, but Coventry wasn't exactly the dream team, was it? I'd been approached by Spurs and Rangers and Charlton. Why would I want to join a struggling club like Coventry?

'Look, Big Man, come and get a few games under your belt. You'll be back in the first team, playing every week, unlike at Wimbledon.

'Forget the medicals. Come and play. I promise you'll enjoy it.'

Looking back, I can now see that phone call saved my career. Gordon saved my career. Gordon believed in me more than in the scan results.

When I finally did the deal I could feel the stress seeping out of my pores, making room for passion and adrenalin and drive to get under my skin again.

CHAPTER THREE

'I found a lump'

I held Sarah's hand and we walked along the banks of the River Avon. The trees were holding on to the last of their summer leaves. The water lapped against the mossy banks, making a soothing, hypnotic sound. A shard of late-afternoon sun lit up Sarah's face and she looked breathtakingly beautiful. I had one of those moments when you get a lump in your throat and you almost want to cry because, just in that instant, everything in the world is so perfect.

'This feels like the calm after the storm. I think it was meant.'

I was 31 years old, and I felt I'd turned a very big corner.

Sarah squeezed my hand, and we walked on in comfortable silence. She knew what I was saying without me having to spell it out. I wasn't just talking about my move from Celtic to West Brom in 2006. I was talking about the bigger picture. Our relationship, how the two of us had finally moved in together, and how this fresh start felt so welcome and so necessary, even though we hadn't exactly planned it.

I thought about Glasgow and my pulse immediately quickened. The city does that to me, even today. I love the place. It was my home through an incredible string of emotional highs. I thought about them deeply and clearly now. At last, I had time to think and reflect with a clear head on my shoulders.

Joni was born there, my adorable son Joni.

I thought about the first time I saw him. I'd stepped outside the delivery suite to answer my phone to my mam and dad when he came into the world. I couldn't believe I'd missed the exact moment my son was born . . . but then I looked at him. I was completely taken aback by how perfect and precious he was. My irritation melted away and was replaced by an incredible wave of love. I gazed at him for a long time, marvelling at his handsome, miniature features and cap of blond hair. He was simply amazing. Just as I had with Bec as a newborn, I wanted to hold him for ever, wrap my big arms around his tiny little body and never let him go.

As I carried him out of the Queen Mother's Maternity Hospital in Glasgow Royal on 5 January 2003, a biting wind whipped around us. I wanted to hold back the wind and protect my little boy from everything cold and bad in the world, for ever. I promised him I would do my best.

Glasgow holds other joyful memories for me, too. I thought back to the hat-trick I scored for Celtic. It was on 20 October 2001 against Dundee United. You just don't forget dates like that. When the first goal hit the back of the net, I felt my blood bubbling through my veins. By the second, it was boiling and fizzing and surging through me like hot lava. By number three, I was so charged up it was like I had volcanoes and earthquakes erupting inside me.

I scored more than a hundred goals for Celtic in my five years there, and every single one filled me with deep pride and satisfaction and left me fizzing and bubbling for days afterwards.

Being hero-worshipped by some of the most fanatical football fans in the world was an incredible experience too. There is nothing as rousing as the deafening roar of the green-and-white back-up squad. The crowd broke into song when I walked out onto the pitch: 'walking in a Hartson wonderland'. The ground rocked beneath my feet. The sheer force and passion of their support always made the hair stand up on the back of my neck.

Literally thousands of men, women and kids screamed and chanted my name whenever I scored. They went completely wild. 'He's got no hair, but we don't care . . . Big John, Big Bad John . . .' It was unreal. When I scored I made 60,000 fans happy in an instant. It was like switching on a light bulb and brightening up the world. I was just a lad from Swansea, but they treated me like some kind of god. It was unnerving at times but irresistibly addictive too. I gave my all to satisfy those fans. They deserved it, and I wanted to deliver for them as much as for myself and for my manager.

Of course, I met Sarah in Glasgow too. I looked at her now, walking brightly in the Stratford sunshine, and I thought, 'Thank God we have moved on and got this far.'

'I have survived.' That's what I thought that day. 'I have survived.'

Survival. The word triggered bad memories. My thoughts switched to the awful lows I suffered in Glasgow too, the lows I had survived. They crashed to the front of my mind in sickening waves.

Not scoring in my first ten appearances for Celtic. That was a recurring, living nightmare at the time. I was fighting for goals alongside Henrik Larsson and Chris Sutton, a potent pair of strikers. I felt sick at the final whistle week after week. Celtic had paid six million quid for my transfer from Coventry in August 2001, and I was giving nothing back.

I looked at myself in the mirror every morning and gave myself a bollocking. 'You can do it, John. Keep going. Train harder. Get that ball in the net. Prove you're worth the money.' It was hard. The pressure was dreadful. Not scoring was unthinkable. It would be the end. An undignified end.

Gordon Strachan had stuck his neck out to sign me for Coventry, and Martin O'Neill threw me another lifeline when he moved to sign me for Celtic just a few months later, but I wasn't repaying him. I wasn't scoring goals.

Sarah and I sat on a bench beside the river and I let the sun warm my eyelids. I shuffled through the difficult memories in my head. In my mind's eye, they were a pack of cards and I was playing poker, hoping I could sprinkle a bit of magic on them just by giving them the right shuffle. I tried to pull a better one to the front but failed.

A massive pang of guilt struck me, right there on the riverbank. It was so acute I felt I was actually back in Glasgow. I was telling lies, so many lies. I was in pain. I could see my marriage ending. I could see myself driving away from my family home.

My kids, Bec and Joni, were inside the house, and I was outside. I was actually locked outside and my clothes were in black bin-bags. I was never going back. Where was I going? What the hell was I doing? They were aged just two and five.

I stared into the depths of the River Avon and I remembered waking up in a new bed. Every morning I went though the same torture, thinking I was in a hotel room, then realising this was my new home, my new bachelor pad in Glasgow.

I relived what I had done and the guilt grabbed at my throat. I'd met Sarah. We'd fallen in love. And I'd had an affair. Every morning it was the same. As my brain caught up with my body, I remembered. My duvet became a thick iron blanket of guilt, weighing me down. I didn't want to get up. I couldn't get up some days.

I was 30 years old and I was suffering a breakdown. Christmas Day 2005 was one of the worst days of my life. Sarah had gone to stay with her parents in Fort William. We were trying to cool things down, but it didn't work. It added to my pain, because I missed her like mad.

'What are you doing, Big Man?' Gordon Strachan asked after I'd dragged myself unwillingly to an early game of five-a-side at Celtic Park. By a happy coincidence, he had become my Celtic manager after Martin O'Neill's departure earlier that year.

'Nothing. I'm on my own,' I shrugged.

'You're very welcome to spend the day with my family, John.'

It was a typically generous offer, but I couldn't impose.

My mate Giovanni, who ran L'Ariosto restaurant in the city until recently, phoned me and asked me to call in. It turned out he had prepared me a Christmas dinner for one. I took it home in a box. It even had a little pot of gravy.

I caught a glance of myself in the mirror above the fireplace in my new home. I'd moved into an incredible penthouse apartment. It cost £2,000 a week and had all mod cons. Plasma televisions, fancy coffee machines, you name it. But what was the point? It felt like an empty prison cell. 'This isn't you,' I thought when I stared blankly back at my grey reflection.

I sat on the huge cream-leather sofa I'd bought. It was big enough to seat six or seven, and I perched uneasily in the middle, feeling marooned, all six foot two of me. I turned on the TV. The *Only Fools and Horses* Christmas special was on, so I watched it for a bit and then looked at the dinner in the box, wondering what I should do with it, when I should heat it up. Eventually I ate the food without tasting a thing, and I cried for my kids. My tears splashed onto the glass coffee table as I held my head in my hands.

I thought of Bec and Joni playing with their toys, surrounded by family and old friends in Swansea. It was what we always did. It was where I should be. It was where I wanted, deep in my heart, to return one day.

Now, I looked up at the blue canopy of sky above the River Avon. The sun was so bright it blinded me. I closed my eyes and I saw flickering images projected onto my red eyelids.

Birds were gliding back and forth along the riverbank.

I thought about Bec and Joni and I let myself slip back in time again. In my mind's eye, they became two and five years old again. It was like watching them through a kaleidoscope, trying to focus, trying to work out what was happening to these two small people who were dancing and laughing and asking me for piggybacks.

I squinted. The poise and height Bec had developed in the last few years had fallen away. She was a tiny, giggling little girl who preferred horses to athletics, and Joni was a wide-eyed toddler, grinning and waving and saying, 'Daddy, look at me!' as he pulled silly faces.

The kaleidoscope in my mind twisted and turned as I allowed myself to watch the memory and tried to focus on it. My children got smaller still. They became two dots in the distance, shrinking away from me as I walked backwards down a driveway, waving and smiling back at them. They disappeared through a shiny front door that slammed shut behind them. The thud made me wince and shudder, and I turned away.

My arms dropped heavily to my sides and the smile slid off my face and landed with a slap on the wet pavement. That's how it felt. 'Keep walking, Big Man,' I said to myself. 'Don't cry, not here.' I quickened my pace. The tears came anyway. I wiped them away, but they didn't stop flooding from my eyes.

I went on autopilot. I dumped my hire car and boarded a flight from Cardiff back to Glasgow. I cried for the duration of the flight. Strangers stared, but I didn't look back. While I cried, I thought about what I had done.

My affair with Sarah had been exposed in the press in September 2005. A Sunday newspaper had finally caught me and splashed the story all over the front page, where it stayed for weeks and weeks.

Now I was in a bachelor pad on my own. There were no photographs on the walls, no toys strewn on the rug or beakers of juice left half drunk on the kitchen worktop. There wasn't even a tin of beans or a packet of biscuits in the cupboard.

The memory made me squeeze Sarah's hand tight, like a little boy not wanting to get lost. We walked to a country pub along the river.

Sarah had been thinking too. It was her turn to squeeze my hand.

'All we need now is a baby,' she said softly as we sat down with a pint and a glass of white wine and a couple of bags of salt-and-vinegar crisps.

My heart swelled. I loved this woman so much. She had never complained. She had given up a life she loved in Glasgow to be with me. She had never questioned why we hadn't conceived for month after month. There was no blame, no bitterness, no self-pity.

'Let's make that IVF appointment, John,' she said. Her eyes were sparkling. I felt so proud to have her on my arm.

'Let's do it,' I said. We'd been together for several years now and had talked about it often enough.

I had lost count of the number of times Sarah had rushed home from Boots with a pregnancy test in a carrier bag.

'Wish me luck!' she'd say, skipping to the bathroom.

Last night the familiar scene played out. I was watching the snooker on the telly. In the silence between the shots, I heard Sarah ripping open the box inside the carrier bag and closing the bathroom door.

'Good luck, babe!' I shouted. As I did, the black rolled beautifully into the top pocket. This is going to be the lucky one, I thought. If someone had offered me odds on this being our lucky day, I'd have staked a packet.

I had looked around our home.

I was sitting in the centre of our open-plan living room. The house was in a stunning setting, built in a private enclave of just four luxury homes, hidden behind electric gates in the picturesque village of Hockley Heath, just outside Solihull. It had the design and feel of a super-sized log cabin. There were huge windows everywhere looking out onto beautiful mature trees and shrubs, and I felt like I was cocooned in the middle of a lush forest. It was safe and homely and slightly decadent all at the same time. I loved it. It would be great to have a baby here. It would be great to have a baby with Sarah.

Minutes later, I heard her padding across the wooden floor in her socks. I turned to face her and her chin was glued to her neck, waves of blonde hair trickling down her face. 'It's another no-no,' she said. She bit her lip but somehow managed to curl up the corners of her mouth. 'It will happen, won't it?'

'Course it will, babe. Course it will.' It had become a depressing pattern, and even though we both put a brave face on it, the monthly disappointment was taking its toll.

Now, sitting together by the river, we raised our glasses.

'Let's do it,' I said.

'Here's to IVF,' Sarah said. The chink of the glasses rang out crisp and clear as a bell. This felt so right. My shoulders softened, and I realised the decision to go for IVF was a relief, not a disappointment. We could break the depressing pattern, do something positive, instead of just hoping and having our hopes dashed every month with that word I hated: 'negative'. We were both so sick of that word.

I thought how our lives had changed. In Glasgow we partied like there was no tomorrow. We 'ripped it up', as Sarah would say. We flew off on luxury holidays to Dubai and Bermuda and we drank bottles of champagne at Gleneagles.

How life had changed. Now we preferred walks by the river and country pubs to living it up in city-centre wine bars. We went out for leisurely lunches, and in the afternoon, instead of reaching for the third or fourth pint, I'd be reaching for the newspaper.

The baby talk made me think about our sleeping arrangements. It hadn't helped that Sarah and I weren't actually sleeping together. I had started snoring really, really badly. It was so bad I kept myself awake, let alone Sarah.

She had got a good job as an art teacher at a pupil referral unit in Coventry, helping teenagers with behavioural difficulties. It was a demanding job, and one she'd done really well to get after quitting her teaching post in Glasgow to relocate with me. Not getting enough sleep just wasn't an option for Sarah. She was up at 6.30 or 7 a.m. to go for a run before work, and she needed to be completely on the ball all day.

The kids she was teaching called her every name under the sun, yet she had to engage them and keep her patience and, above all, try to help them focus and learn through art. It sounded like a bloody nightmare to me, but Sarah loved it.

Sometimes she went out running at lunchtime too, to pound off a bit of stress. She had run half-marathons before I met her. I admired her for that. Of course, my actual job required me to keep fit, but at this point in my life I absolutely hated training.

I would never have voluntarily gone out running, I always hated running. It didn't seem right that I was the professional sportsman yet I had less motivation than Sarah.

'I'm not being funny, John, but I'm just not getting enough sleep with your snoring,' Sarah had said a few weeks earlier. 'It's not good for my health to keep missing out on sleep. It's OK for you, you can sleep in the afternoons after training, but I can't.'

I couldn't argue. I'd taken to sleeping most afternoons, sometimes for hours on end. I surprised myself by the amount of sleep I needed, and Sarah had commented on it several times, questioning how I could possibly be so tired.

'I think I've just got into a bad routine.' It was the only explanation I could come up with. I certainly didn't feel ill or anything, just tired.

'Well, I'm sorry, but I'm moving into another bedroom.'

I knew Sarah's mind was made up. She has this way of looking you right in the eye, and you know she means business. There is never any beating around the bush with Sarah. I admire that quality, and I certainly couldn't argue. She didn't need to say any more, but she did.

'John, you sound like a mechanical digger. It's not even normal snoring. It's just so loud it's absolutely impossible to sleep with you.' Her forehead was wrinkled with worry.

Luckily we had six bedrooms and Sarah chose one down the corridor and made it her own, hanging her art on the walls and adding some pretty lights and fancy cushions. I was left in our old room, which felt like an empty hotel room without Sarah's perfume and clothes and, well, just her presence. It wasn't healthy for our relationship, and I hated not having that closeness you get from sleeping together and waking up together.

On the Saturday night after we'd made our decision to go for IVF, I really didn't want to sleep in separate rooms.

'Can't you just stay in my room tonight?' We'd had a Chinese takeaway and a bottle of champagne. I love champagne and didn't need an excuse to crack open a bottle of Dom Pérignon. Just celebrating spending a Saturday night alone with Sarah was good enough for me. 'You don't have to get up for school tomorrow.'

'I still need to sleep,' she groaned. 'And if I'm going for IVF I need to be in tip-top health. It's all right for you. You only wake yourself up from time to time. But what about me? You can't expect me to lie there all night listening to that row!'

I didn't realise how bad it had become, or how long it had been going on for. Sarah apologised for being so blunt, but I told her not to worry. She was right. I had a problem, and it needed to be sorted out. She wasn't angry with me, just with the situation we were in.

That night I lay in bed alone, feeling a bit sorry for myself, and I thought about something else. I thought about another 'problem' I had. It was one I had never really allowed into my head before, even though I knew it was knocking about somewhere. Suddenly it was rapping its knuckles on my brain, as if to say 'remember me'. I tried to push it away. I tried to sleep. But each time I woke myself up snoring the other problem was jumping up and down, asking for attention.

It was the first thing on my mind when I woke the next morning. I heard Sarah come in from her run and put the kettle on. I felt absolutely knackered, but I lifted myself from my bed and went and sat at the central island in the middle of the ground floor of the house.

'Since we're talking about medical issues, I've got some lumps,' I said to Sarah. I'd first noticed them when I was playing for Celtic, but I ignored them, hoping they would go away.

'What? Where?' Sarah asked the questions baldly. She is not a drama queen. She likes to know all the facts before she makes a judgement. I love the way she deals with problems, and her reaction encouraged me to talk openly.

'Well, on my right ball, actually.' She put down the bran flakes packet and asked me to show her. 'There,' I said, peeling back my black cotton boxers and doing my best to display the offending right testicle.

'I can't see anything, John.'

'Well, you have to dig around a bit . . . I think there are two. One is bigger than the other. Look – can't you see that?'

I had to admit there wasn't much to show, and sitting there in the cold light of day without the nagging thoughts of the night in my head, I could hardly feel the lumps myself, let alone see them.

'Go and see Kevin,' Sarah concluded. She is very vigilant about health. She visits the GP to check out absolutely everything that is not 100 per cent as it should be. She'd had a harmless cyst successfully removed from her ovary a few years earlier, and her attitude was very black and white. 'If there's something wrong, see the doctor and deal with it.'

I am the opposite. I hate doctors. It's not that I'm embarrassed of having to strip off. I've spent my career showering and sharing dressing-rooms with other men. I'd just prefer to let my body sort itself out. I don't like a fuss if I can get away with it. I'd had colds every year practically non-stop through the tough winters in Glasgow. I never swallowed a pill or saw a doctor. Why would I? I always got better in the end.

Sarah was standing over me with that steely look in her eyes. 'Look, if I hadn't had that cyst removed, I'd probably still be worrying about it. What's the point? It was just a lump of skin that shouldn't have been there. This is probably the same. Go and put your mind at rest.'

'OK, I will go and see Kevin.'

'Good. And while we're on the subject, I think we should see the GP about your snoring. It's not normal. It needs sorting out. I don't like sleeping without you.'

We both smiled. 'Agreed,' I said.

It took me a few weeks to get round to seeing Kevin, the West Brom team doctor. It was his job to tend to the medical needs of the players so he was always available, but I put it off for as long as I could get away with before Sarah would nag.

She had taken it upon herself to make an appointment with the GP about the snoring, so I knew that would definitely happen sooner rather than later.

'Next Thursday, 5.20 p.m,' she told me one morning. 'And Kevin?'

'Er, next Tuesday after training.' I couldn't put it off any longer. He was a private doctor. I could have seen him with five minutes' notice if I'd wanted.

During training on the Tuesday, I ran through what I was going to say. 'Look, Kevin, it's probably nothing, but can you take a look at this? I'm sure it's not serious, but you can't be too careful, can you?'

When I actually walked into the medical room at the Hawthorns, I felt a bit like I was going for an interview. I was nervous, and I wanted to get my words right. I didn't want to cause a fuss, but nor did I want to play things down so much he'd dismiss my concerns out of hand. I guess all I really wanted was reassurance.

In the end, I think my side of the conversation went something like this. 'Er, lumps on me balls, mate. Can you take a look?'

Kevin told me in no uncertain terms that I needed a second opinion, and I think he even said he would book an appointment for me so I could have a thorough check-up.

'Yes, doc,' I said, pulling up my shorts and bolting for the door. I had no intention of going for another appointment; I just wanted to get out of there fast.

'And . . . ?' Sarah asked when she got in from work.

'What?' I answered. 'Oh, that? Kevin said everything is fine. Nothing to worry about. No problem at all. Good news, eh?'

'Fantastic! What'll I cook for our tea? Fancy some tagliatelle?'

I sank into the sofa and said 'yes' to anything Sarah said that night. I was just glad the ordeal was over. It was over in my mind. I'd seen Kevin. I'd done my bit. He hadn't diagnosed me with anything horrible. I stopped my thoughts going any further. I convinced myself I'd been reassured. I felt fine. I certainly didn't feel ill. I had no obvious signs of illness – no sickness or diarrhoea, no pain or even mild discomfort. So how could there be anything wrong with me?

When Sarah went to bed, I stayed up watching Sky Sports. I helped myself to a couple of beers and a few sausage rolls, and tucked into a bar of chocolate and a bit of ice cream. I'd been training hard. I'd had a tough day. It wasn't like I was playing for Arsenal and getting put on the scales twice a week. I'd run my balls off for Celtic and it was actually a relief not to be in the first team, on display and under pressure week in, week out.

Things had started off well at West Brom. I scored twice during my debut against Hull and each goal gave me a terrific buzz. I felt a fabulous warmth from the Albion fans, too. They made me feel very welcome, but I've got to be honest: scoring in front of just 20,000 fans didn't give me the plugged-into-the mains feeling I got at Celtic. Nevertheless, I did feel I was playing for a special team in a special part of the world, and I think that feeling was fuelled by my personal experiences off the pitch.

The Midlands felt like a safe haven in comparison to Glasgow. Sarah and I could have a meal in a country pub and push a trolley round Sainsbury's without fans asking for my autograph or without fear of being verbally abused by Rangers fans simply because of the club I played for.

I was anonymous.

We'd had an idyllic start to our life in the Midlands. Well, it was idyllic in theory. It began with a phone call from my mate Stephen Purdew.

'Got yourself a place to live yet, John?' he asked.

'No, still house-hunting as a matter of fact. Got any ideas?'

'Stay with us for as long as you like.'

Stephen owns the Champneys chain of health spas and he was offering us an indefinite stay in the Springs Health Resort near Ashby.

Sarah shrieked with delight when I told her the news. 'What a treat!' she laughed. 'Who gets to actually live in a health spa? It'll be a blast.'

I was thrilled by her reaction. She had lived in Glasgow for 20 years after leaving her parents' home in Fort William. We both enjoyed the spoils of the city. It's a truly cosmopolitan place, and we lapped up the nightlife, the fantastic shops, the rich mixture of people and the whole vibe of the place. We knew the Midlands would be sleepy by comparison, so staying at the plush Springs would be a welcome stepping stone as we made the adjustment.

We weren't disappointed. Sarah giggled when we pulled up in my Audi. I'd worried about how she would cope with the culture shock of leaving Glasgow, but she was shining with excitement.

'What'll we do first?' she said, taking in the surrounding parklands and lakes and the stunning glass facade of the building.

We ate organic salmon and fresh strawberries for dinner, drank champagne in the bedroom and planned which treatments we'd have the next day. For Sarah it was reflexology and a facial, while I was going for a full-body massage.

'This is unreal!' Sarah laughed as we pulled on matching white fluffy bathrobes over our swimsuits and padded down to breakfast in slippers emblazoned with the spa's logo. Another feast awaited us. The breakfast buffet was groaning with fresh fruit, muesli, organic juices and cereals I'd never even heard of.

'Er, doesn't look like there's much chance of a bacon roll in here, does it?'

'It'll do you good, John. You could do with trimming down a bit. Make the most of it.'

And for weeks and weeks, we did. I trained in the gym every morning, even though I just felt like lying on a lounger by the pool, we house-hunted in the afternoons and had fabulous organic meals every evening. My head felt clear, and being constantly with Sarah in this bubble-wrapped world gave me time to think about us and our future.

My divorce had cost me £1.5 million and I'd had to sell my million-pound apartment in Spain to cover it. I was left with a couple of properties and a very large maintenance order. I'm not very good with maths, but even I could work out one simple sum. I was earning £20,000 a week at West Brom. I was 31 years old. It might be the last club I played for, and then what? The money would run out, or at least be vastly reduced, but my outgoings would keep going up.

I had Sarah to provide for now, too. I wanted to marry her and have babies with her. To me, having kids together is a natural part of any loving relationship. I couldn't imagine not having children with Sarah.

'Ta-da! What d'you think?' Her face appeared in silhouette as she blocked the sunlight streaming in through the glass wall of the spa at the Springs. Next I saw her hands waving like a magician. Squinting, I saw she was showing off her freshly manicured nails. I took hold of her left hand. A wedding ring on that hand would be perfect. 'We'll get married soon, I promise,' I said. 'Thanks for sticking by me.'

I hadn't planned what I was going to say next, but I looked Sarah in the eye and made a promise that came straight from my heart.

'I am not going to gamble away big money ever again. This is a fresh start.'

Sarah sank into the lounger beside me, looking like a weight had been lifted off her back. She had never nagged me about my gambling, and we hadn't discussed it for a long time. After all, it was my money. But I knew that she wanted me to cut back, especially if we were going to get married and hopefully start a family together. We'd talked about marriage and babies so many times before, but while my life was in turmoil in Glasgow it had seemed like a far-away dream. Now it was within touching distance, and I didn't want anything to spoil it.

Sarah bent over and kissed me on the cheek. 'Let's have an engagement party,' she said.

'I mean it about the gambling,' I said. She just listened as I went on. 'I have been doing a lot of thinking. I have always said I could stop if I wanted to. Whenever my dad nagged me and told me to get a grip, stop wasting my money, I always said: "Why?"'

'He'd say to me: "Why are you paying a driver £300 to take you to the races in a limousine? Why take £5k with you – why not £50 and go in a cab?"'

'I always said: "Dad, I can afford it. I enjoy it. Nobody suffers or goes without because I gamble. Why do I need to stop?"'

'Well, I am going to prove I was in control all along, because now I can't afford to gamble big money, it's as simple as that. I want to give you the best lifestyle I can. I will never see my kids go without. The gambling stops now. It's over.'

Sarah's eyes filled up. 'That's great,' she said. 'That's really great.'

That night we started to dress for dinner, as we had done for months. The sumptuous restaurant was waiting for us downstairs, but I really didn't fancy yet another beautifully presented, healthy organic meal.

'D'you know what, I could murder a kebab,' I said, flashing Sarah a sideways look.

'You read my mind!' she said. 'Shall we?'

We giggled like a couple of school kids as we skipped out of reception and drove into the night, raiding the local takeaway and stocking up on Discos, Coke, bottles of wine and Mars bars at the all-night Tesco garage.

We ended up staying at Springs for three months. It is a wonderful place for a relaxing spa break, but by the end of our extended stay we felt like inmates in a mental asylum, shuffling around in our robes and slippers.

I'd been paid an £8,000 relocation fee from West Brom, and I spent £1,500 of it on food and treatments at the Springs. It was a once-in-a-lifetime experience, but one I wouldn't rush to repeat. Thanks to Sarah encouraging me every morning, I did make use of the gym, though, and I was raring to go when training started at West Brom.

'I've got every confidence in you, John,' Bryan Robson told me. 'We want a return to the Premiership as soon as possible. You can help us. Just do your best.'

Bryan inspired me. I had been taken on to help bail out a sinking ship. It was flattering, and I wanted to rise to the challenge. I felt like a powerhouse on my debut, against Hull. Sarah was watching the game, and I wanted to impress her. When I scored twice I could have cried. It wasn't until after the match that I realised how much stress I had put myself under.

Bryan hadn't set me any goal targets; he had merely asked me to do my best. But my relief at scoring made me realise I had put myself under a tremendous amount of pressure to prove myself and succeed.

My fitness had been criticised in my last season at Celtic. I remembered the words 'Fat Hartson' booming from opposition fans in the crowd. I also remembered finding graffiti daubed on the front door of my flat in Glasgow saying the same thing. I felt so embarrassed.

My weight *was* an issue. I was more than 18 st., bigger than ever before, but I didn't admit it was a problem on the pitch. 'My size is an advantage,' I said. I can hear myself now, talking away the problem over a pint and a game of cards with my mates. 'I can block players, I can charge in for headers and tackles and other players get out of the way, like they do for Rooney.'

People sometimes did a double take when they saw me out drinking. I could see them thinking, 'He's a professional sportsman – what's he doing?' It pissed me off. I worked hard. I trained hard. I enjoyed a couple of pints, just like my mates back home did when they knocked off from taxi driving and laying bricks.

I thought about how my weight had crept up. At night, when my marriage was ending, I couldn't sleep. 'This is a lie,' I thought. 'I can't lie in my own bed.'

One night I got up at 4 a.m. My heart was racing. I felt flushed with nerves. I opened the fridge and pulled out a can of Coke and a Mars bar. I swigged the Coke and scoffed the chocolate greedily. I wanted to feel better. I needed a sugar rush. Next I opened a six-pack of crisps and started working my way though it. I had to do something with my hands. More Coke. A sausage roll. Eating distracted my mind in those horrible, lonely hours of the morning, when I felt like an intruder in my own bed.

It became a recurring pattern. I did it again and again, stealing down the stairs, guilty steps taking me to the fridge, helping myself to whatever I thought might wash the guilt away for a bit. One night I was so tired out I fell asleep on the sofa downstairs. I woke with a jolt. I don't know how long I'd been there, but it was long enough for a half-eaten Twix bar to have melted in my mouth and dribbled down my chin.

I cleaned myself up, but I didn't really feel clean for a very long time. Guilt stuck to me like a layer of thick grease. I felt sick to the pit of my stomach, and the horrible feeling stayed with me for a very long time as I went through the torturous process of getting divorced.

Celebrating my two-goal debut at West Brom, I'd felt a rush of clean air blowing through me. I remember it clearly. The black-and-white Albion shirt on my back felt like a new skin. I'd shed a lot of the guilt, but not all of it. I don't think you ever shed it all.

After the match I wanted to hug my kids, but, of course, they weren't there.

I thought back to the first time Bec and Joni came to stay at our new house in Hockley Heath. I did the 300-mile round trip to Swansea to collect them twice a week, feeling grateful they were just a car journey away, not a plane ride.

We kicked a ball in the park and tore into pizzas at Frankie & Benny's. Bec told me proudly about how well she was doing with her piano lessons and Joni excitedly explained how he liked rugby now as well as football. I ruffled their hair and drank in their laughter. When I took them back to Wales I cried, just as I had on my return flights to Glasgow.

I bawled my eyes out as soon as I turned the corner of their road. When I stopped at the first set of traffic lights I looked down at my jeans, and they were already soaked with tears.

I cried in Sarah's arms when I got home. 'My kids won't see their daddy before they go to bed. I should be there. I should be reading them a bedtime story. I should be waving them off before school.'

Sarah held me. 'You're living with so much guilt, John; it can't be doing you any good. You're a loving father. You dote on your kids, but you're a professional footballer, too. You have commitments to the club, and you are doing the best you can to fulfil your responsibilities to the club as well as to your children.'

I didn't listen. 'At teatime I should be there, teaching Joni how to use a knife and fork. I should be watching Bec practise her dancing and running. I don't feel like a proper daddy any more.'

'Perhaps you need counselling? This guilt is eating you up. You're living with an unhealthy level of stress and guilt, John.'

'Me? Counselling?' I laughed uneasily. 'I don't think that's quite my style. You know me, I can sort myself out, and I will. I'll do it for you.'

I took Sarah's hand and ran my finger over her engagement ring. Our engagement party was imminent, and I was determined to be the man she fell in love with, the man she used to describe as a 'walking party'.

Sarah threw her arms around me. 'Good,' she beamed. 'Now that's more like the John I know and love.'

A few months later, we threw the engagement party at our favourite restaurant, L'Ariosto in Glasgow. When Giovanni welcomed us that night I remembered his kindness in making me that Christmas dinner a couple of years earlier. I shook his hand and felt flooded with gratitude. I was in a far, far better place than I had been that Christmas, that was certain.

Sarah looked absolutely stunning. I wanted to pinch myself and make sure this was really happening to me.

I was singing 'Delilah', thinking I was Tom Jones. Walter Smith and Alex McLeish, the Rangers managers, were sending over champagne. Sarah was showing off the twinkling diamond engagement ring we'd chosen together in a pretty Stratford jewellers. I hadn't formally proposed. Marrying Sarah was an inevitability we had both felt for a long time.

There was a moment during the evening when I wanted to press the stop button and hold on to the feelings inside me. There was a lull in the conversation, and I sat back in my chair and soaked up the atmosphere. In that instant I felt absolutely great, better than I had in years. I wasn't thinking about football, I was just thinking about Sarah. She was my life now. Sarah and my kids and my family: they were what mattered.

After I'd been at West Brom for just four weeks, Bryan Robson lost his job and was replaced by Tony Mowbray, who left me out of the team.

While Sarah was enjoying her teaching job in Coventry, keeping fit, flitting into Harvey Nicks in Birmingham and relishing the leisurely lunches we had by the River Avon at the weekend, I was sinking at work. I bottled things up for a while, but eventually I moaned to Sarah. 'It's like a vicious circle,' I said. 'All the time I'm out of the first team, my fitness is falling. I can't keep up with the 22 year olds. I'm not the same player I was at Celtic.'

Sarah sympathised and tried to encourage me, but whatever she said, I came to the same conclusion.

'Maybe it's time for me to hang 'em up.'

'No, John, you'll feel so much better when you lose some weight, I'm sure of it.'

Sarah didn't give up easily. She had made the appointment at the doctor's about my snoring and she told me she intended to ask the GP about my weight, too. When we sat in the doctor's surgery, I felt a bit like a naughty schoolboy, being told off for having my hand in the biscuit tin.

The GP's diagnosis was rapid and simple. 'If you lost a couple of stone, the snoring might improve. Being overweight is the main cause of snoring. I could send you to a sleep clinic and there are operations we can do, but I would recommend you try losing weight.'

I sighed. I'd spent my working life watching my weight. I hated watching my weight, but I did it for football. Now I just didn't care enough about the game.

Eventually I wasn't even on the bench, and Tony Mowbray was clearly reading my mind. I was a Championship player on a Premiership player's wage. I was turning up just for the money – £20k a week – and that was something I had never done in my life before. It made me feel terrible, and I also felt trapped. I had huge outgoings because of the divorce and so I had to see out as much of my two-year contract as I possibly could.

Finally Tony Mowbray decided to loan me to Norwich. I delivered the news to Sarah with a deadpan expression on my face.

'Tell me how you feel,' she said. 'I want to know what's going on in your head.'

I took a deep breath. 'How do I feel? OK, seeing as you are the future Mrs Hartson, I will tell you straight.

'I am pissed off with football. I am going through the motions at West Brom. I've worked my balls off all my footballing career and I don't want to do that any more.

'I'm overweight and I'm hating the training. I'm not motivated and I'm finding it incredibly hard.

'I'm just turning up for the money now, and I don't want to be that sort of player.

'I want to see my kids more. The travelling and saying goodbye to them is killing me.

'I want more kids with you, and now this whole divorce nightmare is finally behind me, I want us to get married.

'I love you, Sarah. I am so proud of you and your job and your sunny outlook. I want us to be settled and happy together.'

Sarah looked nervous. 'What's the solution?'

'I'm going to see out my commitment with Norwich, and I want to work out a way of moving closer to my kids.

'The fact of the matter is, when the football isn't right, nothing is right. And when I'm not seeing my kids, everything is wrong.'

CHAPTER FOUR

'I'm coming home, Dad'

'Look! There's a blue cross! John, I'm pregnant!'

I felt the same electric storm sparking though my body that I experienced when scoring goals.

'Come here,' I smiled as I scooped Sarah in my arms. 'That's incredible! That's fantastic! I really can't believe it – let me see!'

We both gaped and smiled at the bright-blue cross for ages. It was almost as if it was going to morph into a beautiful gurgling baby before our eyes, then reach out and hug us. This was going to change our lives. It was something we'd wanted for years, and something we had almost given up hoping would happen naturally.

It was Friday night. Sarah had driven over to Norwich after finishing work in Coventry. She joined me at the De Vere Dunston Hall, a fabulous hotel where I stayed while I was on loan to Norwich.

Life felt good, better than it had in a long while. I was glad to be away from West Brom and I liked Norwich. My cousin Mark had brought Bec and Joni over to watch my debut against Bristol City, and I gave Joni my effort-drenched shirt after the match. I felt a twinge of sadness as well as pride as I handed it to him. He was five years old and he was giggling with excitement at having watched his daddy play in a proper big match. It was great to see, but I knew in that moment that he would never see me play for Wales. As a player

I was on the way down, not up, and that hurt. It hurt a lot.

Sarah came over every weekend I was in Norwich, and we ordered room service, went out for lovely meals and relaxed in the hotel spa. She could have stayed with me full time if she'd wanted to, but that's not Sarah. She absolutely loved her teaching job, even if she did long to start a new career as a mum.

I remembered our early conversations about trying for a baby together. 'To be honest, Sarah, I thought I was done with babies. I thought my nappy-changing, buggy-packing days were over.'

'Well, you were wrong, John! I want your babies. I can't imagine not having your babies.'

'When you put it like that, how can I refuse?'

I wanted Sarah to have my children. It felt such a natural step for us, and being one of four children myself, I was delighted by the thought of having a large family. Maybe we'd even be lucky enough to have two kids together? Then I'd be a father of four, just like my own dad. The thought thrilled me.

I loved Sarah so much. I loved that she wanted my children, and I desperately wanted to give her what she wanted. We didn't imagine we'd have any trouble conceiving.

When I saw her unpacking a familiar Boots carrier bag that Friday night and disappearing into the marbled hotel bathroom, I didn't comment.

After months and months of talking about it, we had finally booked our first IVF appointment for the following Tuesday. In my mind, we had already admitted defeat. The game was up. We needed medical intervention.

I looked at Sarah walking into the bathroom with a breezy 'wish me luck' smile on her face. Poor Sarah, clinging on to the last shred of hope. I felt like a little piece of my heart was thrown out every time another one of those pregnancy kits was discarded. For Sarah, I think it was much worse, because she didn't already have children.

She had soaked my shoulder with silent tears many times. 'Is it me, do you think it's me, John?'

She picked over the fact she'd had that cyst removed from her ovary years earlier in Glasgow, searching for something to blame.

'I very much doubt it's you, Sarah, you're fit and healthy. Maybe it's me. Maybe it's because of my weight. Or maybe it's nobody's fault. Maybe we just need to keep trying, give it time.'

Somehow she managed to piece her heart back together every month, rebuilding hope, smiling again, only to see it torn and trampled upon again and again.

Now this small blue cross proved she had been right to keep on hoping. I hugged her tight. 'I guess we'll have to cancel that IVF appointment!'

'Yes, pity!' she joked. 'I'd booked the day off work!'

We roared with laughter together. I touched her stomach. My third child was in there. The world was turning, whatever my next move at work might be.

I relived the scene in my head when I was on the hotel golf course a few days later. Sarah was in the Midlands, back at work. I was in my last week on transfer to Norwich. Jim Duffy, the manager who brought me in, had left, so I was being sent back to West Brom after just a month.

It was November 2007, and the trees were bare in the surrounding parkland. I allowed myself a little fantasy. When our baby arrived, it would be the height of summer. The trees would be green and lush and the sun would be shining. We wanted a little girl, and in that moment I sensed we'd get one.

'Joni is my boy,' I'd told Sarah. 'I hope it's a girl.'

'I hope so too. I've always dreamed of having a pretty wee girl with blonde curls. I'm so excited!'

I wanted this so much too. I pictured Sarah with a gorgeous baby girl and for the first time ever the image was crystal clear. I could envisage it becoming a reality. I stood rooted to the spot, contemplating the white ball at my feet and the wide, open green in front of me. A thought occurred to me. I could hit this ball anywhere I liked. I could whack it in a tree and lose it for ever. I could roll it into a bunker and have to scrabble around in the dirt to get it out. Or I could do what everyone expected me to do, and try my best to get it in the hole, or as near as can be.

It was entirely up to me. The thought was liberating.

I thought about my career, my life. I hadn't always made things easy for myself, that was a certainty.

The gambling. The brushes with the law. The headlines. Berkovic. My divorce. Especially my divorce. It had made me physically as well as emotionally ill. I was just starting to realise that now, as I emerged from the other side of it and started looking to the future.

Until this point in my life, one thing had stayed constant despite my personal troubles: my football. I always loved my football, no matter what. I always played every game just as I did as a kid at Lonlas, running my legs off, dripping in sweat, willing to smash though a brick wall or jump a ten-foot fence to score a goal if need be.

I thought about returning to West Brom and the sky started closing in. My eyes felt heavy in their sockets. The cold wind pushed at my skin. It seared through my nostrils and ears, scraped down my throat and chilled my heart and belly.

'I'm not enjoying my football,' I thought. Football used to make the sun shine in my sky whatever the weather. Now I felt frozen to the core, so numb I was ice-cold inside. I wasn't just not enjoying my football: I was actually hating my football. I didn't want to push myself physically any more. I was nearly 19 st. I hated running and training, but most of all I hated being left out of the first team.

The first time it happened I treated myself to a Chinese and a couple of pints of beer in the week, just because I could. Now I was doing that all the time. I would never admit it, even to Sarah, but my eating was out of control.

Why did I have to keep doing this? Why couldn't I go home to Wales with Sarah, live near Bec and Joni, go to the Halfway pub for a pint with my mates without feeling guilty, and do something else for a living?

I thought about the dark days when the children first moved back to Wales and I was still playing for Celtic.

Gordon Strachan was very good to us senior players and always gave us a few days off mid-week. The other lads headed off to Gleneagles for massages and saunas, golf and quad biking with their families. Afterwards they all looked rested and were raring to go.

I can still hear Gordon's Scottish growl loud and clear now. 'I've just given you two days off and you look knackered, Big Man!' he snapped. 'The other guys are running rings round you!'

It was true. I was worn out, mentally and physically. I ached to see my kids. I couldn't function without them. Without them I felt physically weakened, like my limbs had been amputated and my energy sapped.

I spent my days off flying to Wales and back to be with them as much as possible. No wonder I was so knackered, but it was worth it. When I hugged Bec and Joni tight after a week apart, I felt instantly rejuvenated, like their energy had poured into me and made me function like a normal human being again.

I took them out for tea and we played in the park, watched videos and went for a swim at the Towers Hotel or the Marriott in Swansea. We all slept in a double bed together, and when they fell asleep I looked at their perfect little faces. They were both beautiful, the most precious little people in the world. It made me cry just to look at them.

Bec's neat school uniform looked so out of place on a hanger in the hotel room. A little girl should be in her own bed on a school night. I knew that, and I wondered what I had done.

We had breakfast in the hotel. The poached eggs, fancy pots of jam and neatly pressed linen napkins were no treat for me. Weetabix in a familiar bowl and tea in my old 'Top Daddy' mug would have been heaven. I dropped Bec at school and wondered what to do with Joni. I wasn't used to being on my own with him all day long. I was used to being part of a family. We kicked a football in the park for hours, then picked Bec up from school and took her horse riding.

'TGI's or the Harvester for tea, kids?' I asked brightly.

'TGI's TGI's!' they clapped. The claps echoed around inside me. I felt hollow. And then they were two little dots, holding hands, going through the black gate and walking down the path to their mum's house. Them waving, me pretending to smile while waiting to turn and cry.

I didn't have to do that any more. I had thanked my lucky stars that I was not having to fly from Glasgow to Cardiff to see them any longer, but the reality was that I was now driving long distances to see them instead. I clocked up 30,000 miles on my Range Rover in my first year at West Brom, and I didn't even want to play for West Brom any more. It was madness.

I'd always wanted to get my coaching badges, maybe even go into management. Why couldn't I do that? What was stopping me? The divorce was finalised and everything was settled in terms of maintenance, so I knew where I stood on that score. It was the right time for change.

I thought of the money I'd wasted. Trickles of guilt and regret seeped through my veins. I scratched my palms nervously. I'd lost countless thousands gambling. Countless. I cringed when I recalled how my agent had had to step in at one point and take control of my finances.

It was when I was at Wimbledon, and it was deeply embarrassing. He had to pay off the bookies for me and set me a budget like I was a little boy getting pocket money. I winced uncomfortably at the memory, but thanked God he had.

Now I didn't have the multi-millions I could have stashed, but I still had plenty of money. I certainly had enough to pay my bills, take very good care of my kids and honour my commitments to my ex-wife.

And I also had enough to relocate with Sarah and our new baby.

I hit the golf ball hard, gave it my best shot. It made a satisfying 'clack' sound as it sailed away from me. It took me a few moments to see where it had landed. It wasn't where I expected, and I shrugged.

You never really know what the future holds, but I was ready to find out.

Packing up and driving back to Hockley Heath when my loan to Norwich ended, I remembered something Gordon Strachan once said to me: 'The fire inside you will go out some day, Big Man.'

I threw the sentence around my head. I hadn't believed it when he said it years earlier. When I was in my 20s I could never have imagined that day coming, but now I knew for sure it had arrived. Gordon had been right. When it came to football, I had no fire left in my belly.

'What's up?' Sarah asked when I pushed open the front door with my large black suit carrier. Before I could reply, I caught a look at myself in the hall mirror. My skin was the colour of rain-clouds and my eyes were dull and hooded. I shocked myself.

'Aren't you pleased to be home, John?'

Sarah looked amazing. There was no bump yet, but I could tell just by looking at her she was pregnant. A low, orange beam of sun had pushed through the clouds and was bouncing off the large plate-glass windows surrounding our living room. Sarah stood in the middle, shining, glowing. There was a magnificent bunch of yellow flowers behind her on the dresser, and from the doorway they framed her face. She looked like a beautiful painting.

'The fire inside you will go out some day, Big Man.' I smelled roast potatoes, and the delicious oily, doughy smell reminded me of my childhood, eating Sunday roasts around the dinner table with Mam and Dad and Big James and Hayley, plus Victoria propped up in the high chair. I felt suddenly homesick for Wales, but very glad to be back home with Sarah.

'Of course I'm pleased to be home!'

I meant it. Being home was what made me happy. Not playing football, not any more.

I suspected West Brom knew that before I did. They had dropped me from the first team months and months earlier. I hadn't been in Tony Mowbray's squad since February, when we beat Cardiff one–nil. It was a hell of a long time to wait around feeling like a reject, trying to keep myself fit and motivated.

I had to face facts. I was struggling to cope. I had lost my willpower. I had no desire to get back into the side. My fire hadn't just burned out; it had been soaked in ice-cold water. I wasn't fit to play, mentally or physically.

I sat down on the sofa quietly. Sarah sat next to me.

'So why aren't you smiling? Aren't you happy?'

'I've said it before, and I'll say it again: when the football isn't right, nothing is right.'

There was a long pause. Sarah knew there was more to be said, and she gave me the space to find the words.

I took a slow, deep breath, scratched at the whiskers around my jaw and said bluntly: 'I'm sick of life.'

Sarah's forehead creased very slightly, but she stayed poised and focused. 'Right. Let's hear it. Tell me how you feel and let's see if we can fix it.'

I felt the knots in my shoulders loosen a little as soon as Sarah spoke. I knew she wouldn't judge me or belittle me or criticise me. I knew she wouldn't try to talk me round either. She had never interfered with my football.

'I just can't go on with West Brom. I want out. The thought of training makes me feel ill. I want to curl up in a ball, not run around kicking one.'

Sarah stroked the back of my hand and listened intently.

'I don't want to play football at all. I am not one of those guys who will go on and on and play for lower and lower clubs, all for the love of football.

'I've been playing since I was a kid, and since the age of 16 my life has been ruled by it. I've lived by some of the hardest training schedules in the world, competing against some of the toughest players in the world. I've been told what to eat and when to eat it. I've been told when to run and for how long and how fast. I've lived by the whistle and the stopwatch. I've been told when I can have a drink and when I have to sleep and where I have to fly to and what I have to wear and even sometimes what I can and cannot say. I've had enough.'

'OK, John, I am going to play devil's advocate here. There are people out there – your mates in Swansea included – who would say you have had the most privileged life, a life most men can only dream of.

'They would say you don't know how lucky you are, and they would say you are whinging and feeling sorry for yourself, and you should pull yourself together and get on with it.

'Are they right? Can't you just pull yourself together? Won't this pass, just like you got over all that trouble with the failed medicals?'

I shook my head slowly. There was a long silence before Sarah spoke again.

'Well, even if you don't want to play football any more, surely you want to keep fit, look after yourself?'

I sat very still and remained tight-lipped.

'Look, I'm a teacher, yet I still get off my backside and run and keep myself fit, not because I have to, but because I want to. It's the right thing to do.

'You're going to be a daddy again soon. I need you to be fit and healthy for us. I don't care what you look like, John. I will love you no matter how big you are. That's not why I'm saying this. I'm worried about your health. At least take more care of yourself?'

As Sarah spoke, I could feel a word forming in my head. It was a dark and ugly word, and I didn't want to say it out loud. I didn't want its murky blackness to spill from my mouth for fear it would leave indelible stains on our lives, our world. To this day I can't remember if I actually spat it out, but as I stuttered about feeling 'down' and 'blue', it was clear to us both what was happening to me. I was suffering from depression.

Sarah didn't flinch. 'Why don't you see the doctor? Maybe you just need a bit of professional help? It can't do any harm, John.'

I stared at the floor and didn't reply. In my head, I thought: 'No. I am not talking to counsellors or taking medication to cure myself. I brought this on myself. It's the backlash from the divorce. I've created this blackness. I've caused my kids to live hundreds of miles away from me. It's my doing that I have to wave goodbye and watch them disappear time and time again. It's up to me to deal with it on my own, face it like a man. I don't need doctors to interfere.'

'Would you move to Swansea with me, Sarah?'

A tear ran down my cheek. Sarah caught it with her little finger and smoothed it away.

'It's killing me not seeing my kids. I can't describe it, Sarah. It's a living hell. It's eating me up from the inside, crippling me in every sense. Being with my kids, being a proper daddy to them, that is the cure I need.'

Sarah was cradling her stomach with both hands now. She wasn't yet a mum, but I could tell she already understood those magical, powerful feelings parenthood brings, the ones that bind you to your kids like invisible ropes. She would have preferred to live in Glasgow, she never made a secret of that. It had been her home for 20 years and she had a great circle of family and friends there.

But still, she nodded. 'We'll do what's best for everyone. You'll see; things will work out.'

Over the next few weeks, I gave up all pretence of trying with my football and fitness. I ate packets of crisps and bars of chocolate if I wanted them, and I watched sport on telly or went to the golf driving range instead of training if that's what I felt like doing.

I was gambling again too, though I kept the finer details from Sarah. She knew I was still betting a bit, and she even came to the races and the dogs with me from time to time. I was careful to only take £300, and we'd spend £100 of that on the meal.

'If I can't beat you, I'll join you,' she said reluctantly. Sarah would never have told me what to do with my own money, though she always kept a beady eye on the budget.

One day, when Sarah was at work and I was alone in the house, I found myself picking up the phone to the bookies and staking £1,000 on a horse. It stoked my belly, firing it up with the familiar feelings of excitement I knew from scoring goals and landing big wins of old.

The horse lost its jockey, and I lost my £1,000, but I told myself it was money well spent. I had passed hours alone in the house without thinking about how much I hated West Brom, or how much I ached to be with my kids. I didn't sit and stew, I had a bit of fun.

West Brom released me from my contract in January 2008, six months early. I'd scored six goals in twenty-four appearances. We had a meeting, and I got the confirmation phone call when I was playing golf at Knowle Park. I grabbed at two words and devoured them: 'early' and 'release'. It was like being let out of jail, and I felt like doing cartwheels across the 9th hole.

I phoned my dad, trying to subdue my delight, because I already knew what he thought.

'Couldn't you extend your career, go down the leagues, play for enjoyment, son? You're only 32. Isn't it too early to retire? You've got a good few years left in you yet.'

I can't remember how many times I'd heard that, and I wasn't in the mood to pick over my many reasons again.

'No, I'm coming home, Dad. It's decided. Sarah has agreed to move to Swansea. Our baby will be born there. I can pick up my kids from school like other dads. I won't have to drive a 300-mile round trip to see them for a few hours here and there. I can't wait.'

'But what will you do, John? What will you do for a living?'

I groaned silently to myself. That was typical Dad. He'd built up his own successful business refurbishing fire extinguishers and could afford to take his foot off the gas. Yet he still worked as hard today as he did when he was grafting to feed four kids and living on a council estate.

'I'm going to do my UEFA coaching badges and think about getting into management. I've got a bit of work lined up with Setanta, too,' I told him. 'I like the telly work, Dad. I've already commented on a good few games, you know, and I love it. I like to chat; I know my stuff. It'll be great.'

And that is how Sarah and I found ourselves driving one way down the M5 one very bright morning in May 2008.

I looked in the rear-view mirror of my black Range Rover at the expanse of motorway falling behind me. 'I can't believe we don't have to drive back,' I said. 'I never want to commute to see my kids ever again.'

As we got closer to Swansea I felt as if huge weights were being lifted off my shoulders. Invisible hands were throwing them away on the motorway behind me. I was almost light-headed with delight. I described the feeling to Sarah and she burst out laughing. 'I'm glad you feel lighter!' she said.

We both looked at her bump, and I burst out laughing too.

Sarah was seven months pregnant. Her swollen abdomen was bulging against the seat belt, the knot of her belly button straining through her white cotton shirt. She was bursting with life. We both were. I felt happy and expectant. I paid my fare on the Severn Bridge and drove across it feeling like a king returning to his realm.

The palace we had chosen to live in was a modern five-bedroom, three-storey house on a very pleasant but unremarkable road in Neath, surrounded by other houses and three houses away from my cousin Mark and his family, who are very close friends.

It cost just £320,000, a lot less than the house we'd left behind in Hockley Heath, ready to be rented out. We could have afforded a country pile, hidden behind gates and set in acres of land, but I'd been there and done that.

'I want my kids to have playmates up and down the street like I did when I was growing up. I want them to be able to walk over to the park and just be normal. I want a family room with a breakfast bar and a dinner table. I don't want a huge polished dining table with twelve seats around it. What's the point in that?'

I'd repeated that mantra over and over again as we house-hunted, and Sarah completely agreed. Our checklist was to be close to Bec and Joni, have enough room for them to come and stay regularly, not to be too far from my parents and siblings, and basically to have a warm, comfortable family home where the people we loved would feel welcome.

'Have we done the right thing?' Sarah asked when we finally collapsed on the sofa, packing boxes stacked up all around us.

I looked out of the living room window and across the hills piled up on the horizon.

I imagined Bec and Joni coming into view. They were black dots, but instead of disappearing over the horizon they were walking towards me, getting closer and closer until I could see them clearly, smiling and waving.

'Definitely,' I said to Sarah. 'Most definitely.'

CHAPTER FIVE

'I'm the luckiest man in the world'

'I haven't felt this good in a very long time,' I said to Sarah.

My job with Setanta was going really well. It had started with me commentating on the odd match here and there, and when I'd finally left West Brom in January 2008 I did more and more shows.

'Work till the end of the season, John, and we'll give you a contract,' said Colin Davidson, the boss, and he was true to his word.

It was music to my ears. I was absolutely loving the work. I'd always been happy to put myself in front of the camera when I was a player, chipping in my thoughts about the match. Now I was being paid to do it, and I found it came very naturally to me.

Next week I was flying to Glasgow to report on an Old Firm match between Celtic and Rangers, and Sarah was booking in with the local GP and fixing herself up with a midwife appointment.

The first time I'd sat in the commentary box at Celtic Park I was flooded with nostalgia. I saw myself on the pitch in the familiar Hoops green-and-white shirt with my number ten on the back and I felt very proud, remembering the glory days. But I didn't want to turn back the clock.

I didn't have to train. In the mornings I could have a bit of breakfast with Sarah and just enjoy being an ordinary partner, an ordinary dad. I could pick up Bec and Joni from school, take Bec to her athletics and watch Joni play football at the weekend.

I travelled up to the Old Firm match the day before, kissing Sarah goodbye before catching a flight from Cardiff to Glasgow. I had a spring in my step and I felt excited.

Now I was spruced up in a Hugo Boss suit, crisp white shirt and salmon-pink silk tie. I was in a warm commentary box drinking a cup of tea, watching the match from the best seat in the house. I felt like a million dollars.

I was commentating on the game with my mate Terry Butcher. We had worked together on loads of matches and sparked off each other well. He was an ex-England international and an ex-Rangers centre-half – the perfect foil to an ex-Wales international and an ex-Celtic centre-forward.

We had a leisurely couple of pints the night before the match and a fantastic steak dinner at the Glasgow Hilton. All the talk was of football. Systems, players, managers, tactics, fans, transfers: we discussed them all, and I loved it.

When I sat in the studio the next day and the lights went on, I felt like a switch had gone on in my head, lighting up some of those dark corners that had blackened my mood for so long. I felt alive, buzzing, like my old self. I felt the same blood-rush I felt when I was in the dressing-room before a big match, about to go on the pitch and run my legs off.

Now I didn't have to run, I just had to talk. It came easily to me, and the punters seemed to like what I did. 'You nailed it, Big John!' the first text to the show said. 'Spot on, Big Man – exactly what we were saying at home. Offside, no question.' Terry got the same reaction. We were both successful, but there were never any egos clashing. I think that's why it worked. We genuinely loved what we were doing and respected each other.

After the game, I was on a high. I tucked into the corporate hospitality, savouring the generous comments and sumptuous food with equal vigour. I was being slapped on the back. Managers and ex-managers were passing positive remarks about me, saying I'd got it just right with the commentary. I felt fabulous when I flew back to Cardiff.

Sarah hugged me tight when I got home. She had just two months to go before the baby was due, and she was clucking round the house like a mother hen.

'I've missed you! Well done! I'm so proud of you, John. 'Can I get you something to eat? You must be tired? You looked great on the telly, really great.'

I was pleased she thought I looked great, because the truth was, I felt heavy in my jeans.

'What have you had to eat?'

'Oh – you know, a few fancy sandwiches after the show and I picked up a burger at Glasgow airport, but that was hours ago . . .'

I stopped there. I didn't want to list everything I had eaten. I'd had a McDonald's at Glasgow Airport and a couple of packets of Pringles with some Cokes on the flight. Before the match, I'd had a fry-up in the hotel: four rashers of bacon, a couple of eggs, two pork sausages and a few rounds of toast. I couldn't have a growling stomach when I was live on air. I'd eaten a Kit Kat I picked up at the service station when I got petrol coming out of Cardiff Airport. I'd probably eaten more in 24 hours than most people do in a week. I was treating every day like Christmas Day, and I just didn't want it to stop.

'Shall we order a takeaway, then? Chinese sound all right? I'm avoiding curry because of the baby . . .'

'Great, sounds great to me.' I didn't have to train tomorrow. That was always my justification. In fact, I didn't even have to work until a mid-week match in four days' time. I twisted the cap off a cold bottle of Beck's and took a long drink. I was in heaven.

My media work gave me the confidence boost I needed to finally get my act together and work hard for my coaching badges. I discussed it with Sarah and she was delighted. It was something I'd always planned to do when I retired, and my TV success made me believe I really had it in me to pass on my experience to others, and maybe even be a manager one day. I booked myself in for the training sessions for the first of the three badges.

'You know, John, it'll be great for your health, too,' Sarah said as she helped me get organised. I had to buy new shorts and tracksuits for the course because none of my old ones fitted me. Sarah didn't beat around the bush. 'It's supposed to be me bursting out of my clothes, John, not you! I don't want to burst your bubble, but remember what that doctor said in the Midlands?'

Her words made me falter. I immediately thought about Kevin, the West Brom doctor. 'You need to get this checked out properly.' That's what he'd said when I told him about the lumps down below.

I thought about my lie to Sarah. 'There's nothing wrong.'

The lumps on my right testicle hadn't gone away as I'd hoped, even though it was a couple of years on. If anything, I think they'd got a bit bigger, but you still had to dig around to really see them.

'Don't pull a face, John,' Sarah continued. 'I'm only saying that when we went to see that GP she told you to lose weight, and you haven't. You've gained weight. It's no wonder you're still snoring so badly.

'You really should try to trim down. I've said it before and I'll say it again. I'm worried about your heart giving out. Losing weight will help you with your coaching, too. You need to set a good example if you're going to be teaching others, not to mention the fact you're about to become a daddy again. I can't have you pegging out on me. Agreed?'

'Yes, agreed.' I was actually very relieved she wasn't talking about Kevin and the lumps. I didn't want to talk about that ever again.

I didn't feel unwell, so I didn't think I had anything wrong with me. If the snoring kept me awake, I had plenty of time to sleep in the day. Also, because of my height, I could carry the weight without looking obese. I think that's why I let it get so out of control.

But Sarah was right, as usual. Deep down, I knew I wasn't respecting my body, and I had to lose weight. I knew it was the right thing to do, but my willpower had other ideas. It couldn't stand up to the whispers in my head that reminded me of how hard I had trained in the past, how I had put up with Arsène Wenger's bland rabbit food at Arsenal and the strict training diets at other clubs, and how much I deserved to give myself a break now I was retired.

I loved it when my dad phoned on spec when the sun was still shining in the afternoon. 'All right if I call round?'

We sat in the garden, chatting and eating and drinking. Simple stuff, but for me it was a big deal. I was a free man. I could enjoy a beer and a burger with my dad without a care in the world, and it felt great. If I fancied a pint over a game of darts or cards at my local, I could do it. I loved that. I don't like being on my own. I'd bought a box at Swansea as much for my friends and family as for myself. I like having people around me, and my friends always filled the box up.

We'd only been back in Swansea for a month or so when I signed my two-year contract with Setanta. My income was a fraction of what it had been when I was playing football, but it was enough. I was home, and I was happy, two things no amount of money can buy. 'I'm the luckiest man in the world,' I said to Sarah one night. It wasn't a special occasion, I was just so happy with how things had turned out. The only blot on the landscape was my size, but that was something I was going to deal with.

I didn't quite manage it before Lina was born, on 14 July 2008.

It's a date I will never, ever forget. I was more than 19 st., and if anything was going to make my heart give out, Lina's birth was it. It was the most terrifying experience I had lived through.

'This is it,' Sarah had announced three days earlier, on the Friday night. 'The contractions have definitely started.'

She'd had a brilliant pregnancy, sailing through without a hitch. When I drove her to the Singleton Hospital that night I didn't expect there to be any problem whatsoever. Besides, Sarah is a tough cookie, and I knew she'd cope no matter what.

Seventy-two hours of labour later, my nerves were snapping, but I still had every faith in Sarah. She was strong and serene. I looked at her with awe, lying in agony on the delivery bed, determination etched on her exhausted forehead.

The baby was finally coming. Our baby was about to be born. Sarah was pushing. I was holding her hand, willing the baby to be born, willing the pain to stop for Sarah, and willing that moment to come when we could hold our baby in our arms. Sarah made sharp white dents in my hands as she dug her fingernails into me.

It was white all around. White sheets. White tiles. White machines beep, beep, beeping. That horrible sterile hospital smell caught in my throat.

'Brow presentation. Emergency Caesarean.' Now Sarah was white and I was suddenly struggling to drag oxygen into my lungs.

'What does it mean? What's going on?'

A midwife hurriedly explained that Lina was trying to come out face first instead of headfirst, which was extremely dangerous. She wouldn't make it unless Sarah had a Caesarean.

The room fell silent. Nurses and midwives ran. White coats everywhere. Flashes of metal instruments, Sarah moaning in pain and fear, then falling silent too.

There was blood on Sarah's belly, and our baby was out, but she was also silent.

I held my breath, waiting for a cry, a murmur even, but there was nothing, absolutely nothing. The only sound I heard was my own heartbeat. I thought my baby girl was dead.

The silent chaos in the room continued. It was silent pandemonium, like watching a silent movie on a screen. Eight or nine doctors were running now, equipment wheeling, but there was still no sound. No swish of coats, no rattle of trolleys. Just utter, terrifying silence.

Our baby was whisked way, still silent. She was floppy too, her fragile limbs dangling like wet spaghetti. Her tiny face was grey and ripped and bloodied: she had fought so hard to break out into the world she'd torn the skin off her cheeks. Sarah watched in utter horror. She looked shattered. Then, finally, it came: a newborn cry.

Our daughter had been silent for two and a half minutes, but it felt like two and a half days.

'Our little fighter,' we christened her. 'Lina, our little fighter.'

It was a full week before we could hold her and take her home. She lay in an incubator with tubes attached all over the place. It broke our hearts, but it swelled them too. Looking at Lina, looking at this tiny scrap of life who had fought so hard to make her entrance into the world, I felt so proud to be her daddy.

When I finally got to carry her out of the hospital and take her home, I felt flooded with relief. Not only had Lina made it, but Sarah and I had made it too. We were engaged to be married. We had a beautiful daughter and a fabulous life.

'To Lina,' we giggled, clinking champagne glasses and cooing over her blonde hair, rosebud lips and pretty blue eyes. Her skin healed quickly and she looked dazzling now, just like her mum.

'You certainly got what you ordered,' I joked.

'I know,' Sarah laughed. 'If I could have designed my own baby, I would have designed her. She is absolutely perfect.'

Lina's arrival reinforced how I felt about all the other changes in my life. I'd been officially retired for six months, and I had absolutely no regrets. I didn't miss playing football, and my work with Setanta was perfect. I looked forward to every match, to wearing the suits and having a few beers with my colleagues the night before. I enjoyed the flights and the banter and the reaction I got from viewers. The hours were ideal, too. I did a couple of mid-week matches and maybe a game or two at the weekend, all within the UK.

Sarah planned to return to work and had found herself a good job in a secure unit in a local school for adolescents and a place in a nursery for Lina. Her start date was January 2009, but as the date drew closer Sarah realised she couldn't do it.

'John, I just don't want to leave Lina,' she said as we packed away the Christmas decorations. 'I adore working, but I just can't leave my baby, not yet. She'll only be five months old. It's too soon.'

I gave Sarah a huge cuddle. In my heart, I was glad. We'd had a fabulous family Christmas. My mam and dad came over, and Bec and Joni, of course. It was like old times. I saw my sister Hayley and Big James and his three boys.

My younger sister Victoria brought over her daughter, Livia, who is a year older than Lina and couldn't stop fussing over her baby cousin. I felt so proud when I saw Sarah holding our baby, in the centre of my home, my world. It's where I wanted her to be, and I felt blessed that's what she wanted too.

'Don't worry, I won't be sitting around doing nothing!' she said. 'First of all I'll help you arrange your tribute dinner.'

I certainly had no worries there. Sarah is a doer, and she's extremely switched on. She has her dizzy moments too, of course. I mean, I can give her directions to somewhere she's already been three times and she'll still get lost. 'Do they give those degrees out to anyone who sticks their hand up?' I'd joke. 'Glasgow School of Art you say you went to. Got a degree? Are you sure?'

She knew I was only teasing. Since our move to Swansea, Sarah had agreed to take full control of all of our finances and give me a weekly spending allowance, just as my old agent had had to in my gambling days. She had found out I'd had a few relapses in my dark moments in Stratford, and we'd both decided this was the best plan of action. I trusted her implicitly to do a great job. I didn't often feel tempted to have a flutter these days, but I didn't want to run any big risks. I think once you've gambled at the level I did, you have to admit it's an addiction.

Now I wasn't earning big money playing football, we simply couldn't afford for me to lose large sums of money any more. I'm not embarrassed to admit that. It's a bit like being an alcoholic: if you can acknowledge you have a problem and stay out of the pub, you're on the right track. For me, having Sarah holding the purse strings removed my temptation. It was a relief.

Sarah threw herself into the arrangements for my tribute dinner in Glasgow. Lots of footballers have tribute dinners back at their old clubs, and it was my turn to have a Celtic tribute dinner. It's a chance to revel in past glories, auction off some memorabilia and generally have a great old knees-up.

'What d'you think of this?' Sarah asked one day when I got home from the driving range. I'd joined Fairwood Park Golf Club and divided my leisure time between escaping up there for a few rounds or seeing my old mates over a pint or a game of cards or pool.

JOHN HARTSON TRIBUTE DINNER
Sunday, 29th March 2009
Hilton Hotel Glasgow
Join a host of top sporting personalities as they honour Celtic Legend Big Bad John at his tribute dinner.
Guest speakers are former Republic of Ireland and Liverpool hero John Aldridge and top comedian Bobby Davro; the compere Rob MacLean of Setanta Sports.

Drinks Reception, 4-Course Meal followed by the above Guest Speakers and a Sports Auction at the end. Dress code is lounge suit.

'Sounds perfect,' I said.

I looked at the words 'Setanta Sports' and wondered if I should mention the rumours I'd been hearing. Seeing as Sarah was our financial controller, I decided I had better keep her fully in the picture.

'You know I got a two-year contract with Setanta and I still have a year to run . . .'

'Yeeesss . . . ?'

'Well, there's talk the company is in trouble. Financial trouble. It could fold. And, contract or not, I could lose my job.'

'Well, we'll worry about it if and when it happens, John,' Sarah said. She didn't flinch at all. 'I have no worries about you. You'll always work. The viewers love you. You tell it how it is and you know your stuff, John. You're priceless. Don't worry.'

The axe fell a few weeks later, and I was absolutely gutted. I totted up I'd been on 187 flights for Setanta, mainly to Scotland. I had a wardrobe full of 50 designer suits.

I'd loved the buzz of being in front of the camera. Each game had been a privilege and a pleasure to commentate on. I felt comfortable in my job, and the feedback I got backed up how I felt about my performances.

I was very disappointed for the others who lost their jobs too. In my heart I knew Sarah was right. My agent had already had calls from Sky and ESPN offering me other work, and I also had my weekly football column in the *Scottish Sun*, but I worried some of the other lads, the ones working behind the scenes, might not be so fortunate.

'Don't worry, John, you always come up smelling of roses,' Sarah said when she caught me frowning. 'You're Big Bad John, for God's sake!'

When we took our seats at the Celtic tribute dinner, Sarah's words rang in my ears.

My Celtic theme tune, 'Big John . . . Big John, Big Bad John', boomed out of giant speakers and my best goals were displayed on a giant screen.

'And it's John Hartson! What a goal. It's John Hartson again. Look at that power . . . ! I don't believe it, he's scored . . . !'

Gordon Strachan stood up and cleared his throat, and the room fell silent. We'd had fantastic performances from all the guests and speakers. Bobby Davro and the comic John Gahagan had us clutching our sides with laughter, but it was actually Gordon who brought the house down, regaling the crowd with tales of my attempts to avoid the dreaded bleep test at training.

'The lads would all take bets on how far John would go to avoid the bleep test . . . I lied once and said we had the test that day. Right on cue, John piped up, "Sorry, Gaffer, I'd love to do this, but I've pulled something in my side . . ."'

The crowd roared with laughter, just as my team-mates had when Gordon had said: 'Only joking – it's not for two days, you'll be right as rain!'

I looked at Gordon and grinned. This man had just made a thousand Celtic fans laugh out loud. He was their hero, and he was certainly one of mine.

We stayed up until four in the morning. I didn't want the night to end. All my family had flown up for the occasion. My sister Victoria made a point of telling me how proud she felt, and my mam's broad smile and moist eyes spoke for her. My dad looked absolutely fit to burst with pride as he shook hands around the room and chatted about 'my boy, my son John'. Sarah looked gorgeous as she floated around looking like she hosted celebrity parties all the time.

I laughed to myself when I remembered how she'd first told her mother we were an item. Her mum, Katherine, is a big Celtic fan and knew my name well, while Sarah didn't have a clue I was a well-known footballer.

'Er, Sarah dear, do you mean *the* John Hartson,' Katherine had said eventually, when she put two and two together. 'He plays for Celtic –. you've actually seen him play! Didn't you recognise him?'

Sarah shook her head. She'd been to the odd game, but she wasn't what you'd call a football fan by any stretch.

'Have you not noticed him in the papers, seen his picture on the back pages?' Katherine went on.

'No, Mum! I look at the news headlines and the horoscopes and then I chuck the paper in the bin. I never look at the sports pages. I wouldn't have a clue what any of the footballers look like. Besides, half the guys in Glasgow will tell you they play for Celtic, and if John had told me that himself I probably wouldn't have believed him!'

I loved that about Sarah. She couldn't give two hoots about the following I had in Glasgow, but she has always been able to handle it like a pro.

'How can you top this?' I thought when I looked around the room at the Hilton. I was 34 years old and I'd had the most incredible career. I looked at Sarah and wondered what would happen next. And I remembered her words: 'You always come up smelling of roses, John! You're the luckiest man I know.'

A few weeks later we took Bec, Joni and Lina to Center Parcs in Sherwood Forest. We booked out the biggest and best lodge available. I felt like really letting my hair down and enjoying myself with the kids.

It was such a pleasure to see Bec and Joni fussing round Lina, taking her under their wing as their new little sister, and I was determined to give all the kids the best possible holiday.

We could have flown off to Barbados or Florida if we'd wanted to, but I'd discussed my feelings with Sarah. 'When I was a kid, we went to a caravan park in Tenby – and you know what, that's what kids enjoy. They don't like queues at airports and blistering heat. They don't like being packed off to kids' clubs or being babysat by strangers.

'Center Parcs is ideal. And then why don't you and me book a break to Dubai later in the summer on our own? We could ask your mum to look after Lina.'

Sarah agreed. She had flown up to Scotland with Lina several times and knew all about the stresses and strains of flying with a baby, so she was in no hurry to take the children abroad.

The Center Parcs break turned out to be a great decision. Even though I was over 19 st., I didn't let my weight hold me back. I was riding bikes, climbing ropes, driving go-karts, playing table tennis, swimming and sliding – you name it. I had Joni on the back of my bike, Sarah had Lina on hers and Bec cycled beside us.

Every evening I cooked a barbecue and sat round the table with my kids and Sarah. I felt absolutely brilliant, and Bec and Joni had pink cheeks and the big, toothy smiles kids display when they are really happy.

Lina was proving to still be the little fighter she was at her birth, babbling loudly and trying to keep up with the older two even though she was still learning to walk. We tickled her and called her Dinky Doo and Iggle Piggle and Ninky Nonk, and she threw back her wispy blonde curls and gurgled happily.

I thought about countries I'd visited in the past. I'd sunbathed on spectacular beaches in Bermuda, one of my favourite holiday destinations, and I'd loved strolling down Las Ramblas in Barcelona when Celtic played in the Champions League. It was the most beautiful city I'd seen.

When I played for Wales, the team was driven under police escort to the best hotels in Düsseldorf, Eindhoven, Zurich, Bologna, Kiev, Oslo, Moscow and Milan. Most of the time I only saw the insides of fancy cars and hotels, but they were the most luxurious, palatial hotels you could dream of, like royal kingdoms.

Even when Sarah and I did fly to Dubai a few months later, in June 2009, I found myself saying, 'You know what, this is spectacular, lying here looking out over the Persian Gulf. But Center Parcs was something else, wasn't it? I think it was the most enjoyable holiday I've ever had.'

Sarah and I stayed at the five-star Habtoor Grand Resort in Dubai. It was truly spectacular. I looked across at Sarah, lying back in the sun, surrounded by white sand and perfect palm trees and distant skyscrapers that shimmered in the heat. It was great to see her relaxing, having a well-earned break from our little fighter girl. Sarah looked a million dollars, and I felt very lucky. She was such a support to me. It was months since I'd left Setanta, but Sarah continued to tell me not to worry, we'd be fine. She'd even enrolled as a supply teacher so she could pick up some work now Lina was getting bigger.

I'd had a few meetings with the BBC in Scotland, and I had a steady flow of freelance pundit jobs on ESPN and the Welsh channel S4C. Sky TV was even talking about me doing a show, and I had lots of radio work on the go. I was also about to complete the last of my three UEFA coaching badges and was looking forward to putting them to good use.

I smiled at Sarah even though she had her eyes shut. She was right. I was the luckiest man in the world. Life was great.

We had started talking about fixing a wedding date, and even though Lina was still only ten months old we were already trying for another baby. After all the trouble we'd had conceiving Lina, we had decided to try almost straight away for another one, and every month Sarah was using ovulation kits and dragging me to the bedroom when the time was right. 'Not again!' I'd complain, before pretending to be forced against my will into bed.

Sarah opened her eyes and squinted in the sun. 'I was thinking about the wedding, John,' she said. 'What if I'm pregnant?'

I was delighted by her optimism, just as I had been delighted by her willingness to try for another baby so soon after having Lina, especially after what had happened at her birth.

'Look, it took ages to get pregnant last time, Sarah,' I said softly. 'The same thing could happen again. I don't think we can plan our wedding around another pregnancy, do you? I think we should just go ahead and do it. Are you trying to wriggle out of becoming Mrs Hartson or something?'

'No way! You're right, John. Let's think about some dates for next summer. But I'm telling you now, if I'm pregnant we'll have to postpone it. As much as I can't wait to be your wife, I'm not waddling round in a wedding dress!'

We laughed our heads off, and when we eventually fell into a contented silence I thought about my own size.

I was 19 st. 3 lb now, my heaviest weight ever. My shorts felt tight and I was actually the one waddling around, but I was still tucking into burgers and chips every day on holiday. I felt tired, carrying round so much weight. I was so tired I was sleeping a lot in the afternoons, but I put that down to the fact I was still waking myself up snoring at night. My breathing sounded very laboured, Sarah said. I felt a bit embarrassed, to tell the truth. All these problems were because of my weight.

I thought about my coaching badges yet again. I'd promised myself I'd be more disciplined and get fit before I finished them, but in fact I'd got bigger and the final one would be completed in a matter of weeks.

'I'll definitely get in shape for the wedding, babe,' I said. 'I promise you that. I'll be a few stone lighter when we get married.'

I wanted everything to be perfect on our big day. I wanted our future together to be perfect, and as I soaked up the hot sun and relaxed, I felt sure it would be.

When we returned home, nothing contradicted how I felt. I completed my 'A' licence – the third and most gruelling of the three coaching badges you need to be a professional coach. Only 12 of us out of 27 on the course passed, and I was delighted with myself. The world was my oyster now. A new phase in my career was there for the taking, and I was looking forward to what the future would bring.

Chapter Six

'I found that lump again'

SARAH

The events of July 2009 will stay with me for ever. What happened was so shockingly unexpected, so emotionally charged and so ultimately life-changing that each twist and turn is etched on my memory and still burns as vividly in my mind today as it did when I was living through it.

I will tell you everything I recall, but, of course, there were times when I had to leave the hospital to look after Lina, and I had to sleep and go to Tesco's and do all the mundane things that stop the roof from falling in completely. Thankfully, John's younger sister Victoria kept a detailed diary so that John would be able to look back and know exactly what had happened to him during his time in hospital. It makes me cry to read some of the things Victoria wrote, but John and I will share extracts from the diary to fill in any gaps in our own memories.

Friday, 10 July 2009 started out as a very ordinary day. As usual, the sound of Lina giggling and gurgling in her cot woke me up. 'Daddy,' I heard her babble, and my mind turned to John.

I sighed when I opened my eyes and remembered there was a big empty space beside me in our bed. John was sleeping in the spare room because his terrible snoring had been keeping me awake lately. He weighed 19 st. 3 lb and our family doctor had told me being overweight was one of the most common contributory factors to snoring. I'd discussed John's health with the GP a few weeks earlier, when I popped in to have Lina checked over, as she had a wee cough and cold.

'It's not just the snoring that worries me,' I found myself saying. 'He's so massively overweight I'm worried about his heart giving out. His breathing sounds very laboured at times, too. It's not right.'

The doctor flicked through her records. 'John hasn't been in for a check-up for ages,' she said. 'Why don't you get him to come in for a medical? We can talk about his weight and his snoring . . .'

'Actually, he's been tired a lot, too,' I added. 'He's been sleeping in the daytime. He used to have a sleep after training, but he hasn't been training for ages. I can't understand why he gets so tired.'

I surprised myself by listing all those symptoms. They had crept up on us and become a part of everyday life for, well, I don't even know how long. Not long at all, I thought, but with a baby to look after I hadn't really had much time to think about it.

John was big and strong and indestructible. That's how I saw him, and that's how he saw himself. Lina's wee coughs and colds were a much bigger priority for both of us at that point in time. She was a dainty 11-month-old baby girl, and John was a powerhouse. Nothing broke him. You never had to worry about him, not really. He'd admitted he needed to get his weight down, and I knew he was serious about it. He'd just finished his coaching certificates and was raring to add a new strand to his career, as a football coach. He acknowledged he needed to be leaner and fitter and said he wouldn't let his weight pull him back. He was adamant he was going to get in shape.

I went with John for his medical. It was all pretty routine. The doctor said John might be able to have an operation on his palate to help control his snoring. He also talked to John about weight loss, and John casually threw into the conversation that he'd had a lump on his right testicle for a while. I knew all about it. John had shown it to me, but to be honest I couldn't see a thing. It certainly wasn't like something you had to push around in a wheelbarrow! John explained to the doctor that you had to poke around quite a bit to actually feel it. I left the room while he was examined. 'Best get it scanned,' the doctor said. 'Make sure it's nothing to worry about. I'll book you in for an ultrasound scan.'

On Friday, 10 July, as I got ready to go for a long-standing appointment in Birmingham, I could hear John's snores right down the landing. They were deep, loud, grunting growls that made me wince. He sounded truly awful. For weeks now we'd tried to make a joke of it, and before he went to bed the night before John had laughed and said with a twinkle in his eye: 'When are you going to let me back in the boudoir then, Sarah?'

'When you stop sounding like a farmyard!' I retorted with a mischievous grin, but deep down I wasn't finding it that funny.

I picked Lina out of her cot and changed her nappy before tucking her into bed with John for a cuddle, as I always did while I fetched her bottle. John looked groggy at first, but his face lit up when Lina waved her favourite fluffy bunny under his nose, held out her squishy little arms and said, 'Want Daddy, Daddy, Daddy!'

'Hello, Dinky Doo,' he smiled, stroking the bouncy blonde curls on the nape of her neck. He sounded very tired, and he squinted quite dramatically when I pulled open the blind to let the bright morning sunshine filter into the room.

'Sorry, Sarah,' he croaked. 'D'you mind shutting that? I didn't sleep a wink. I feel OK if you want to leave Lina with me; I've still got a bad head. Can you get me some more paracetamol . . . ?'

My heart sank a little. How long were these headaches going to last? He'd been like this on and off all week. I scooped Lina back into my arms and carried her downstairs to the kitchen for breakfast.

I wedged the phone between my ear and shoulder as I helped Lina spoon herself blobs of warm Weetabix and banana. I called Louise, our trusty babysitter, explaining I had a lunchtime appointment with the orthodontist in Birmingham and didn't want to strap Lina in the car for hours to take her with me. 'I'll be over in half an hour,' Louise said breezily, and I felt myself relax a little. Louise would stay in the house with Lina while I got my appointment out of the way, and with a bit of luck John would get himself together and feel well enough to take over before I got back around 5 p.m.

I slipped into the spare room to kiss John goodbye and explain the arrangements. 'Are you sure you're OK?' I asked. 'I can cancel this appointment, you know.'

'No way,' he said. 'I'm not that bad now. You go. I'll be OK. I'll sleep it off.'

Fine, I thought. Sleep it off. Get yourself better. I want you back to your normal self. I want my 'Big John' back. I touched my tummy gently. There was no bump there yet, but as I shut the door quietly and left John sleeping, something made me place a protective hand across my belly.

I didn't offer John as much sympathy as I normally would if he was ill because, the truth is, I thought he was still feeling the after-effects of his weekend in Dublin. He'd been to a big Celtic function the previous Saturday and hadn't been right since. I felt a bit fed up that he was all partied out when we had our own celebration to have: we had another baby on the way and I wanted John to crack open the champagne, not lie in bed moaning.

As I steered the black Volvo out of the drive and headed for the familiar link road to the M4, my mind replayed the unpredictable events of the previous week.

John and I had been trying for another baby for eight months. Every month when the blue line failed to appear on the pregnancy test, I sobbed. It wasn't fair. I desperately wanted another baby. Our family wasn't complete, and my hormones were bellowing at me to have another child. I was forced to relive the vicious circle of desperate hope followed by raw disappointment that I'd gone through when we tried for a whole year to conceive Lina. It had been horrendously draining. Trying for a baby dominates your every waking thought, and here I was again, consumed by broodiness and desperation to carry another child.

I'm normally the type of person who doesn't worry about anything until it actually happens. What's the point in living like that? Why tie yourself in knots about a 'what if'? That's what my head told me every month and every day and every minute, but my heart would never listen. It constantly ached with anticipation, and it broke with depressing regularity every time my body didn't do what my heart willed it to.

After so many months of despair, John and I were about to embark on a course of IVF. I cried after I phoned to make the initial appointment. I didn't want to go through all that physical pain and emotional torment, all those injections and drugs and endless hospital trips. But, of course, I would do anything if it meant giving Lina a wee sibling. John supported me wholeheartedly. In fact, he thought I was pretty amazing to want another child so soon after having Lina. He told me he was glad I wasn't one of those women who had one baby and decided it was too much like hard work. He admired my energy and drive and said he felt honoured and lucky that I wanted his children. I admired him, too. He was already a father of three and had been a daddy for a decade, yet he wanted another baby with me. 'I like a big family round the dinner table,' he had told me. I wanted him to have it, I really did. Each time I saw an empty chair round the dining table, I ached to fill it.

I bought two pregnancy tests while John was in Dublin attending his Celtic Football Club function. It was Saturday, 4 July, and he was guest of honour at the dinner at the swanky Citywest Hotel. As he sank a couple of pints of Guinness and prepared to take his seat at the centre of the top table, I was hovering nervously in our en-suite bathroom, looking at the white window on the pregnancy stick laid out on the side of the bath, willing it to turn blue. My hands started to shake and my throat went dry. After so many disappointments, I had already prepared myself for the worst. I was biting my lip, willing myself not to get too upset, not to cry. After all, we had the IVF appointment all booked up. We hadn't run out of chances. There was no need for tears. Lina wasn't even one yet. Her first birthday was ten days away. We had plenty of time . . . 'Oh my God!' I screamed, staring in disbelief at the bright-blue line on the test. 'I'm pregnant!'

I looked at myself in the mirror and did a double take. Was this real? Suddenly, I didn't trust myself or the test. I hadn't been prepared for a positive result. I didn't have John there to look at the test stick and tell me it was actually real. With shaking hands, I tore open the second test and repeated the process, just to make sure I wasn't imagining things. Slowly but very surely, another electric-blue line appeared. I grabbed my mobile phone and clicked on John's name with trembling fingers.

'Hi, babe!' I said excitedly. He was in a noisy bar, enjoying pre-dinner drinks. 'How are you?'

'Fine,' he said. 'Having a good time. Lovely hotel. They're doing a montage of my goals on a big screen during the dinner, how about that? Got a bit of a headache though . . .'

'Had too much Guinness already?' I teased. 'Anyway, you need to swap your pint for champagne,' I joked. 'You've got some celebrating to do!'

It was a bad line, but I heard John cheer excitedly when I told him our news. He sounded delighted and told me he couldn't wait to get home and start the celebrations with me. He would take an earlier flight than planned the next day and be home after his lunch with the Celtic bosses on Sunday afternoon. 'It's absolutely brilliant,' he said. 'I can't believe it!'

'It's early days,' I replied, suddenly feeling protective of the new baby. 'Don't tell anyone yet, John.' As soon as he put the phone down, I knew John would call his mum and dad and word would spread like wildfire around the family. Sure enough, within the hour our home phone and my mobile became a hotline, with family phoning to congratulate us. John never could keep good news to himself. He always behaves like a child on Christmas morning, bubbling over with enthusiasm. I don't know why I ever bother to say, 'Keep it quiet.' It just isn't John's style, and even though I tell him off afterwards, I guess I find it quite endearing.

It was a bit of an anticlimax when John got home. He scooped me in his arms and gave me a huge hug and kiss, telling me how delighted he was about the baby and rubbing my tummy. He didn't look himself, though, and almost as soon as he got through the door he said he had to lie down.

'Still got a bad head,' he apologised. 'I swallowed a strip of Nurofen at the airport, but they didn't help one bit. I've taken the maximum I can every four hours, but nothing's helping. Sorry, Sarah, I need to sleep this off.'

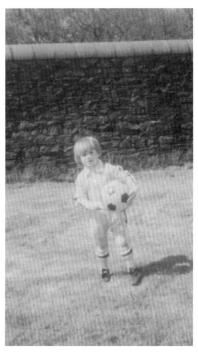

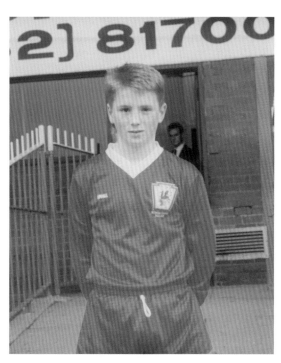

Me aged three and a half wearing my first-ever football kit: a bright-yellow Leeds strip.

Here I am at Dens Park, Dundee, representing the Wales Boys' Club under-14s. Unfortunately, I broke my arm after just 15 minutes of the match.

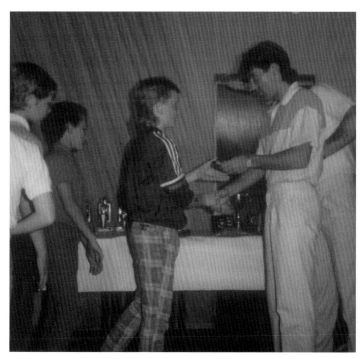

Dean Saunders, one of my heroes and a fellow Swansea lad, presenting me with a trophy at a function for Lonlas Boys' Club.

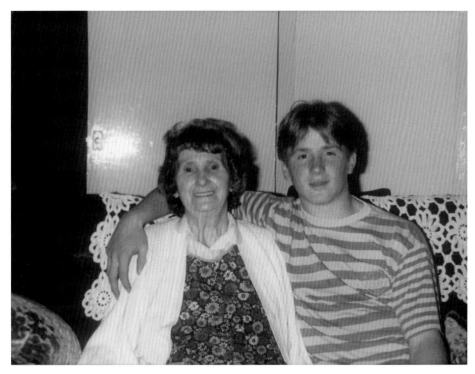

Me aged 16 with my lovely nana Lena.

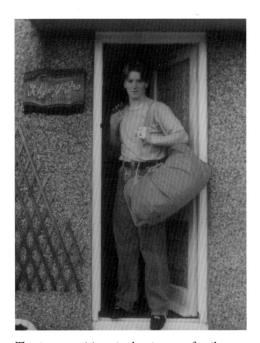

This is me at 16 again, leaving my family home for Luton.

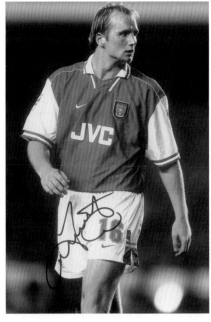

Me in my glory days at Arsenal in 1995.

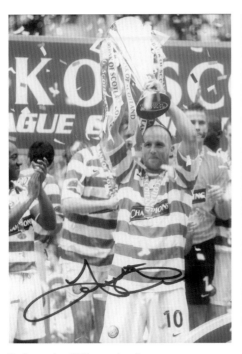

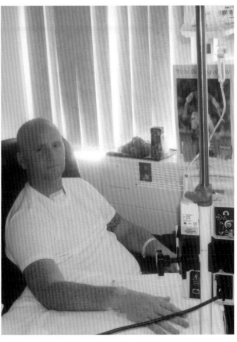

Lifting the SPL trophy for my third and final time in 2006.

Sitting in a chair at Singleton Hospital was all I could do when I came round from my illness in August 2009.

The tens of thousands of messages of support I received from friends, fans and former colleagues and managers gave me a terrific boost.

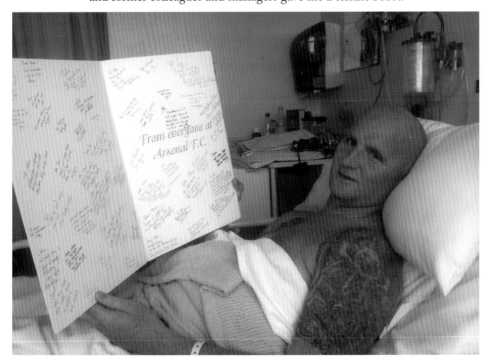

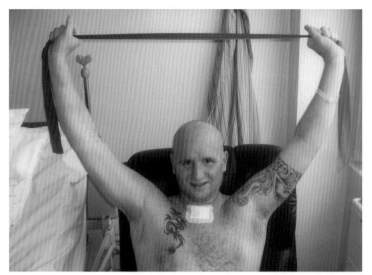

Daily physiotherapy helped me regain my power.

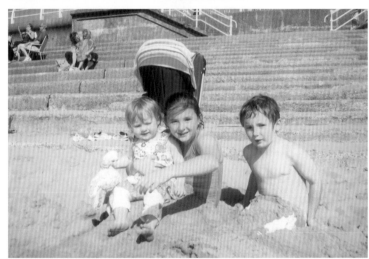

Bec, Joni and Lina on a day out at Aberavon beach in August 2009.

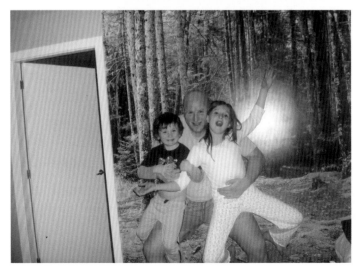

Enjoying Center Parcs with my kids Joni and Rebeca in September 2009.

Chemo made me lose my appetite, but I enjoyed tucking into my favourite pork rolls in Fort William in October 2009.

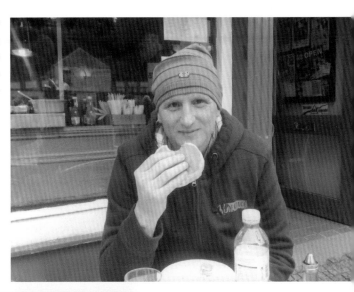

My sister Vic and dad Cyril at a charity function in aid of the John Hartson Foundation in November 2009.

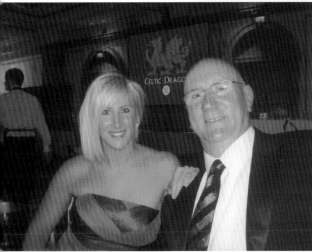

Marrying my beautiful wife Sarah at Neath Registry Office in December 2009.

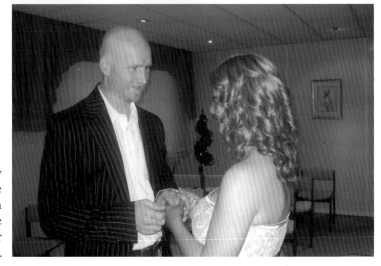

My cousin Mark Hartson and his new wife Joanne were our only witnesses on our wedding day.

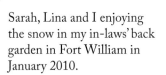

Sarah, Lina and I enjoying the snow in my in-laws' back garden in Fort William in January 2010.

This is Sarah's favourite picture of me and Lina, who is cuddling her favourite 'rabby' toy at home.

Stephanie at three months with big sister Lina in June 2010.

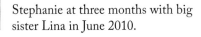

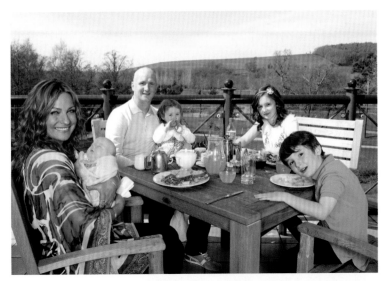

Posing for glossy pictures in *OK! Magazine* with my beautiful wife and my four fantastic kids in June 2010.
(© Ed Watts)

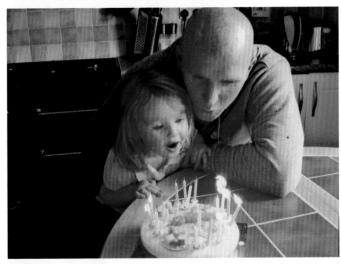

Me and Lina celebrating her second birthday on 14 July 2010, the day I climbed Ben Nevis.

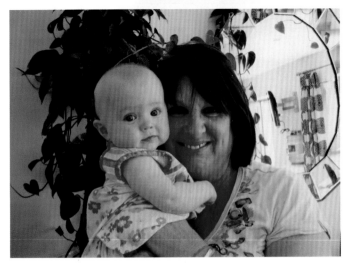

My proud mum Diana and baby Stephanie at home in August 2010.

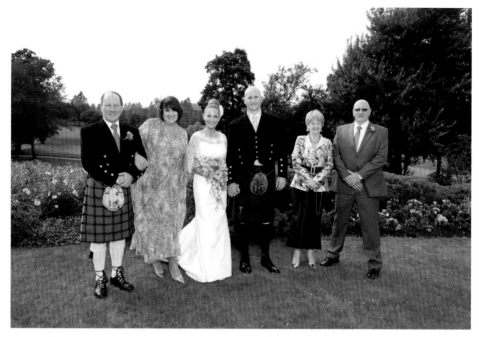

Me and Sarah celebrating our marriage with both sets of parents. Sarah's dad James is on the left next to my mum Diana, and Sarah's mum Katherine is next to my dad Cyril on the right. (© Ed Watts)

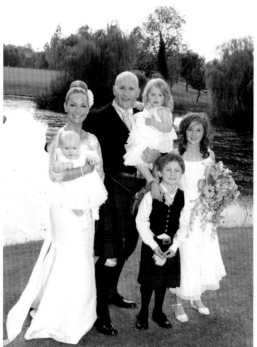

Celebrating my wedding on 23 July 2010 with Sarah and my four kids. (© Ed Watts)

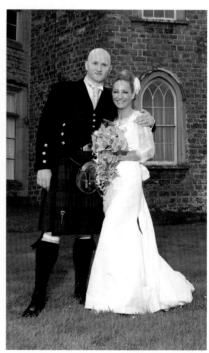

Me and my stunning bride Sarah at our wedding party. (© Ed Watts)

'That's what you get for giving it the big yahoo with the boys in Dublin,' I said, rolling my eyes.

He didn't reply, and I assumed I was right: he had overdone the Guinness, and who could blame him? He had not only spent the night being feted by football bosses and Celtic supporters in a plush hotel, but he'd just found out we had another baby on the way. If you can't get stuck into a few drinks in those circumstances, then when can you? I wasn't going to cause a fuss. I could see that all John wanted to do was try to sleep, and I wasn't going to argue. 'Go on,' I smiled. 'Get your head down.'

I honestly thought John had the mother of all hangovers, so I left him to it and played with Lina on the living room floor, building Mega Bloks and playing peek-a-boo with her teddies until her bath time. I just wanted John to recover quickly so he could join back in with normal life, but it wasn't to be.

He could barely get out of bed the next day, or the day after that. He staggered up to the golf driving range a couple of times, but he wasn't himself at all. He had his hospital appointment on the Thursday, to check out the lump in his testicle. Normally we went together to anything like that, but John was adamant he was going alone. 'It's not worth you coming,' he insisted. 'It's nothing.' I didn't push it. I thought perhaps he was a bit embarrassed and that's why he didn't want me there.

When he came home he looked a bit jaded, but reassured me that the doctor had taken a look at the growth and decided it simply needed to be removed.

'What exactly did he say?' I asked. John muttered something about 'malign'. 'Do you mean malignant or benign?' I asked. I felt I was only getting half the story. 'It's quite an important difference,' I said.

John wasn't sure, and I made a mental note to insist on going with him to the next appointment. He is the sort of person who glazes over and looks for an excuse to get out of the room if someone talks for too long, and I suspected that was what he'd done at the hospital.

'Don't worry,' he said. 'They said they'll send me a letter and that the appointment should be quite soon.'

I thought back to a few years earlier when I'd had a cyst removed from my ovary. It had worried everybody and wasn't pleasant, but in reality it was a harmless lump and a minor operation. I honestly thought John's growth was something similar. Looking back, I wonder if I was in denial too. The warning signs were there, but I didn't allow myself to see the big picture. 'I'll come with you for the next appointment,' was all I said. Little did I know that John was going to need a lot more support than that. Had I had the slightest suspicion about what was about to happen, I would never have travelled to Birmingham that Friday morning.

JOHN

Lying in bed, I heard the front door click shut as Sarah quietly slipped out. It was silent in the room, too silent. I felt guilty just lying there in the dark. I don't like being on my own, and I don't like the dark. It was horrible. Normally I sprang up and buzzed around the house in the morning, playing daft games with Lina, tucking in to mugs of tea and bacon butties at the breakfast bar with Sarah and sorting out the day ahead. No two days had ever been the same since I left West Brom, in January 2008. I hadn't had time to miss playing professional football since retiring from the game. I looked across the room at the enormous expanse of wardrobes lining the wall. Inside I had 50 smart suits, all bought for my new job as a television commentator. I'd been on 187 flights in my first year as a pundit for Setanta Sports. Now just the thought of getting out of bed made me feel shattered. I had no energy at all. My head hurt like mad. It had nothing to do with the booze in Dublin. I didn't want to frighten Sarah; it was best she thought I had a hangover. But I knew the truth. I'd had a couple of pints, a few glasses of wine with dinner and finished with a liqueur or two in the bar. I had been nowhere near drunk.

My head was hurting even before I got on my flight to Dublin. I swallowed handfuls of painkillers at Cardiff Airport, hoping they'd do the trick. I don't normally get headaches, but I assumed a good dose of

Nurofen was all I needed. I didn't want to let anybody down. I was guest of honour at the Celtic function. I knew from experience how these occasions played out. Celtic had invited all their hardcore fans. The manager and chairman would be there, and the committee of the supporters' club. As the 'chosen one' that night, I'd be feted and applauded in extravagant style.

I wasn't disappointed. Arriving at the Citywest Hotel, I was treated like royalty. I was seated in the middle of the top table, and I felt very proud when a montage of all my best goals for Celtic was played on a giant screen. Sarah's phone call about the baby capped what should have been a perfect night. I was so delighted I couldn't help phoning my mum and dad with the news. It was too good to keep to myself, and I wanted the world to know my fourth baby was on the way. Me, a dad of four! It was unbelievable.

Despite the great atmosphere, I wasn't at ease. At times, the headaches made me wince and squint. They were stabbing me down the back of my head and behind my eyes. I swallowed more paracetamol, counting out the maximum dose each time, and one of my mates slipped me a couple of his wife's migraine tablets. Surely they would kick in soon? I tried to focus on the images of me on the big screen in my Celtic kit, hitting the back of the net, but it was a struggle just to keep the images sharp at times. The banter, the fabulous food and the company kept me going, but I was working very hard just to be myself. We chilled out in the bar until 2 a.m. and met for a slap-up Sunday lunch before I flew home that day. I held myself together because I had to, but it wasn't easy.

It wasn't until I sat on the plane home that I had my first dark thought. 'These headaches are unnatural.' That's what I thought. I watched the clouds out of the window and said to myself, 'I just don't need this.' I was relieved when I saw the familiar lights of the Cardiff Airport control tower in the distance. I just wanted to get home, see Sarah and Lina and go to sleep. It never occurred to me for a single second that the headaches might be life-threatening. I mean, who thinks a headache is going to kill them? As we landed, I pushed the dark thoughts out of my head. Yes, the headaches were unnaturally bad, like nothing I had experienced before. But I wasn't going to panic: it's not my style. Taking to my bed was as bad as it would get. That's what I thought as I lurched into a broken night of sleep.

I woke at 6.30 a.m. the next day with an even worse headache. I couldn't believe it. This was getting boring. I told Sarah not to worry about me and to do her stuff with Lina and leave me to rest, even though I hate being on my own in the house. Whenever Sarah is out, I don't know what to do with myself. Normally I'd fix up a round of golf or a game of pool or darts with my mates if I found myself at a loose end. I never just stayed in on my own.

I prised myself slowly out of bed and shuffled to the kitchen. We have a magnificent view of the Neath hills out of the back of our house, and the light was streaming in through the window. I recoiled in shock when it hit my face. My eyes stung, and I held my head with both hands as a massive wave of burning pain reverberated around my skull. I phoned the doctor and asked for an appointment. 'Bad headaches,' I told the receptionist. I felt a bit embarrassed. It sounded petty and trivial. I mean, who goes to the doctor with a headache? I certainly never had before, but I knew this was different.

I drove myself there in absolute agony. It was all I could do to concentrate on the road in front of me and navigate myself up the path and into the doctor's surgery. By this time, any embarrassment had disappeared. I was just desperate for help. I did my best to articulate my pain. 'It's so bad it's just mind-boggling,' I think is how I described it. I was told to carry on taking painkillers. I was given a prescription for a box of sachets of painkillers to dissolve in water, but they didn't have any effect at all. I don't blame the doctor for not picking up on my symptoms earlier, by the way, and she is still my GP today. We are all human. She prescribed what she thought would help me, but unfortunately they didn't. Sleep was my only release, and I was glad to get back home, collapse into bed and close my eyes.

I managed to sleep in short bursts, but each time I woke and opened my eyes, the pain hit me like a sickening, dull thud. It got so bad I was suppressing screams and moans. I didn't want to cause a fuss and alarm Sarah. She was flitting around, looking after Lina, and I didn't want to be a burden. 'What will I make for our tea?' she said, popping her head round the door. She's a great cook, and I asked her to make steak and home-made chips, my favourite, hoping I'd be able to sit at the table and tuck in enthusiastically like I usually did.

I felt comforted just knowing Sarah was in the house. She unpacked my suitcase and did the washing, answered the phone and sorted out the bills. I felt guilty, though. She had taken a career break from teaching so she could spend more time with Lina, and yet here she was looking after me too. It wasn't right, and as the hours and days dragged by that week, I felt increasingly frustrated by my body.

I dragged myself up to the golf driving range a couple of times in the evenings. I think I was trying to prove I was OK, even though I was still in agony and couldn't think of anything but how much my head hurt.

Each time Sarah asked how I was feeling I had to admit I still felt 'terrible', and I did in every sense of the word. I was in dreadful pain, and I felt awful for collapsing in a heap while Sarah was tearing round doing everything on her own. She didn't get cross and she didn't complain. She's a trouper, she really is, and she just gets on with things. 'Can I get you anything? Why don't you have a bath, see if that makes you feel any better?' Sarah provided a stream of support and helpful suggestions, and I told her I would be absolutely fine. I just needed to rest and sleep.

I think I did a good job of playing down just how bad I felt. 'D'you fancy going up to the beach and taking the baby in the pram?' Sarah asked one morning that week. 'We could get a bag of chips, get some fresh air? Go up to Aberdovey?' It was something we did together a lot and something I loved. Often I was the one who suggested it, but as I lay there wrapped in my duvet I could honestly think of nothing worse. Just the thought of daylight on my face made me shudder.

'Sorry, no,' I muttered. Sarah looked concerned and nodded quietly.

'OK, babe,' she said. She still thought I'd overdone it in a big way in Dublin and I still didn't want to worry her by disillusioning her. I didn't dare share my deep-rooted fear that these headaches were unnatural, like nothing I had experienced in my life before.

'Just leave me to my own devices,' I said. 'I'll be fine once I've slept this thing off. Sorry about this.'

As the week wore on, I found it increasingly hard to sleep. At night I'd eventually drop off around 10.30 p.m. after swallowing yet more paracetamol, but would wake frequently with crippling pains in my head. I woke myself up snoring because it was so loud. My breathing wasn't right at all. I buried my head under the covers, cradled my skull in my hands and willed myself back to sleep several times through the night. I was exhausted, but when I woke up at 6.30 a.m. the next day I still felt tired out and drained of energy, and my headache was even more blinding than the night before.

When I did sleep, it was fitful. I had dreams and flashbacks. It felt like my life was crashing around inside my head. I had never spent so much time in bed. My head was nailed to the pillow with pain, and it felt like memories and dreams and fears were running riot in my head, taking it in turns to torment and confuse me.

The scan appointment to check out the lump in my testicle came through for the Thursday of that week. I only had to travel down the road to Neath Port Talbot Hospital. I'd drag myself there and get it over and done with. Did I make any connection between the lump, whatever it may be, and my headaches? Not a single one. I mean, we are talking about two completely separate parts of your body. I knew absolutely nothing about testicular cancer, and it never even crossed my mind for a split second that a lump down below could be responsible for the pains in my head.

I wanted to go on my own, even though, with hindsight, it was probably dangerous for me to drive, as I was squinting and my vision was going blurry on and off. Sarah was busy with Lina and everyone was at work in the afternoon. I didn't want to worry anybody, even though, if I'm being very honest, I knew in my heart I was about to get bad news.

I gritted my teeth when the male radiologist asked me to remove my underwear and lie on the bed. He used the same sort of ultrasound wand I'd seen before at baby scans, and I found it very depressing when I looked at the screen. Normally you're buzzing with excitement, looking for a little face or a tiny foot, trying to see if it's a boy or a girl. Now here I was not wanting to see anything at all. My whole body tensed when I felt the cold jelly on the wand touch my skin. I wanted to be anywhere else but there. It was a huge inconvenience. I remember my head pounding as I looked at the small white lump that clearly showed up on the black screen as the radiologist examined my right testicle. There was a second, smaller lump alongside it, too. I can't remember the exact words he used, but when the words 'testicular cancer' eventually filtered through to my brain I just froze. 'We will write to you with an appointment,' he told me. I didn't ask any questions at all, I just wanted to get out of there as quickly as possible.

I assumed it would be an appointment to remove the lump, or even my testicle. I wasn't ready to take in all the gory details. All I wanted to know was that the offending growth would be removed and that would be the end of the problem. I shed a few tears driving home and reached for my mobile.

It was 4 p.m., and I was meant to be in the S4C commentary box at 6 p.m. to cover a UEFA match between Llanelli and Motherwell. It was only eight miles down the road from me, the closest TV job I had ever had to home and one I'd been looking forward to, but I knew there was no way I could get through it.

I had no pain in my testicle or any other symptoms of testicular cancer as far as I was concerned. I just had the terrible headaches that were now stabbing me right in the nape of my neck and making my eyesight wobble.

I phoned the producer. 'I'm sorry, Emyr,' I said. 'I would never normally do this. I've never missed a day's work in my life, but I'm just not well enough to come in tonight.'

'Er, it's a bit late in the day to phone up, John. What's the problem?'

I hadn't even told Sarah I had testicular cancer, and I had already made up my mind not to tell her just yet. It's not something you want to talk about, is it? I wasn't ready to face it, but I didn't want the producer to think I was messing him about. I took a deep breath. 'I'm sorry,' I said. 'I've just been diagnosed with testicular cancer.'

My words hung in the air like a bad smell. I could barely believe what I'd just said.

Emyr nearly broke down on the phone. 'I'm devastated for you,' he said. 'Go and get yourself well, John,' he said. 'Get yourself fit and we'll see you back.'

I put the phone down, shed a few more tears, then drove home in silence. Sarah was unpacking the shopping when I got in. 'I've phoned in sick,' was all I said. I went back to bed and had a truly terrible night. My head felt like it was going to explode with pain. It was becoming intolerable, like a blinding, deafening, grating pain swamping my whole brain. Shutting my eyes brought no relief, and I was slipping in and out of sleep, wondering why on earth I was suffering such terrible headaches when I had just been diagnosed with testicular cancer. How unlucky was that?

On the Friday morning I remember Sarah coming in and out of the spare bedroom, smiling her lovely warm smile and bringing Lina in for a cuddle. I smiled back and said I felt OK, even though my head hurt so much I couldn't see or even think straight. I was relieved when she left me to carry on sleeping, because at least when I was asleep I didn't feel the pain. Yet every time I woke it was still there, more excruciating than ever. 'I've got to sort this out,' I thought. 'I can't cope with this pain any more. I've got to sort this out. I need help.'

I knew Sarah was on her way to Birmingham, so I reached for my mobile and called my sister Victoria and asked her to come over. My mum called in to see me at some point in the morning, too, having heard I was in bed with a 'bad head'. I had lost track of time, and all I can recall is her tiptoeing softly into the room and asking, 'John, love, is there anything I can get you? Anything I can do to help?'

'No, Mam, I just need to sleep this off,' I groaned, shielding myself from the beams of sunlight that framed her in the open door. 'My head's killing me. Is Lina OK? Can you get me some more paracetamol?' I tried my best to sound upbeat. You know what it's like with your parents. You don't want to worry them, do you? Mam was used to cheering me on, proudly watching me on the TV and telling her friends about my latest award or achievement. We were comfortable in those roles. We'd played them out for 20 years or more, right from when I started to shine on the football pitch as a young lad. But this new scenario was alien to us both, with me coiled up in pain, clutching my head, and Mam not knowing quite what to say. It must have been awful for her.

I staggered out of bed eventually. I had the bright idea of steaming my sinuses with Olbas Oil and boiling water in a bid to clear my head and blast out the headache. I knew I was clutching at straws, really, but I snorted greedily at the hot air, desperately letting it sting the inside of my nose in the hope it might cut through the folds of pain packed behind my eyes. It had no effect at all, and the effort of moving downstairs to the kitchen made me feel tired and nauseous. I sat on the sofa clutching my head in my hands and trying to stop my eyes closing over. I remember seeing Lina wander into view with Louise the babysitter. I forced a smile, but it took every ounce of my strength. Lina was giggling happily, wonderfully oblivious to my pain. She was showing me a fluffy bumblebee that sang a song: 'Don't worry, bee happy'. The words flashed up in bright red on its striped belly. I squinted in agony as Lina gurgled and held it up to my face so I could have a closer look.

When Victoria arrived, she tried to chat gently about my headaches to weigh up how bad they were. I sensed uneasy glances being exchanged, but, like me, I think my mum and my sister were still hoping the pain would subside any time now. It couldn't go on for ever could it? I just had a bad headache. I'd been to the doctor's and I was taking paracetamol and resting. What else could you do? Nobody wanted to press the panic button.

Mam and Vic stayed for a few hours, I think, but I found it hard even to make small talk, and eventually I hid back under my duvet, willing sleep to numb my pain. They both agreed to leave me resting for a while, but try as I might I couldn't get to sleep. My head felt like it was going to explode, and before long I stumbled out of bed again and called Victoria on her mobile.

'Vic, I think I need to get to the hospital and sort this out,' I spluttered. My head was banging relentlessly and I could see no sign of a let-up. If anything it was getting worse, and I was reaching the end of my tether.

'I think I've got swine flu,' I said, trying to suppress the clouds of fear building in my mind. It was all over the news at that time, and it seemed the most logical explanation.

'Don't be so daft,' Victoria laughed, slightly nervously. 'I'll be right there.'

I looked up the symptoms of swine flu on my laptop. I was squinting to shield my eyes from the glare of the screen as I searched the NHS website and clicked on 'symptoms'. My eyes fell on the words 'unusual tiredness', 'headache' and 'shortness of breath or cough'. A wave of sickness hit me from nowhere, and I walked to the bathroom and vomited in the washbasin. The fluid was watery and a peculiar dark-grey colour, like nothing I'd seen before. I normally find it difficult to be sick even when my body wants me to be. But this time I had no control. It came from nowhere, and it was disgusting. I didn't want to look at it, and I washed it away quickly.

I stood at the front door in shock, anxiously waiting for Victoria, and when she came in I led her straight to the laptop. She scoured the page too. 'Er, what about the symptoms you don't have, like a runny nose and sore throat?' she asked. 'Honestly, John, I don't think you have swine flu. I don't know what you've got, but I think you need to get onto the doctor again.'

I agreed, and as I dialled the GP surgery Victoria continued surfing the Internet. I assumed she was looking up more details about swine flu. In fact, I found out when I eventually read her diary that she was looking up the symptoms of a brain tumour. I had pretty much all of them, but Vic kept that to herself and never flinched. What a girl.

I explained to the doctor's receptionist that my headaches had got much worse. These weren't just headaches, they were excruciating, throbbing head pains. 'I'll get the doctor to call you,' she said.

A few minutes later, a doctor phoned back and told us to go to the Medical Assessment Unit at Singleton Hospital. She would call ahead and let them know we were on our way.

Sarah was just pulling up outside as we left the house. 'Where are you going?' she asked, looking worried. I could barely open my eyes.

'I can't bear it any more,' I explained. 'My head hurts so much I feel sick.'

Sarah said she'd sort Lina out and follow us to the hospital. Victoria drove. I was beyond making decisions or functioning normally. It took all my strength to hold my head up and breathe through the pain.

I started crying in the car on the way to the hospital. I thought of little Lina, about to celebrate her first birthday. Only the week before, Sarah had talked about the pink cake she would get for Lina, the fluffy and sparkly toys she loved and the friends and little cousins we'd invite over for a birthday tea. I wanted to cuddle Lina and make her giggle, like I normally did. I also thought about Rebeca and Joni. I was a lucky man. Fantastic kids, both of them, aged ten and six years old. What if something terrible was happening to me?

A dark thought descended. I didn't want to leave my kids without a daddy. I wanted to cherish every second with each of my children. And what about the new baby? Sarah was due in March, but suddenly March felt like an impossibly long way off. In that moment I urgently wanted to become a daddy of four, but I felt trapped by my pain and I just couldn't picture myself in the future. I put my hand across my eyes and sobbed. Victoria was as good as gold. It must have been dreadful seeing her big brother crying like that, but she just made comforting remarks, gritted her teeth and drove.

When we arrived at the unit, Victoria dealt with all the rigmarole of booking me in.

'John Hartson. Let me see . . . the last address we have for you is Tyn-y-cae Road,' the receptionist said, rooting through old records. Unbelievably, Victoria and I both managed a little laugh.

'Er, he's moved a few times since then,' Victoria said politely. A few of my old houses flashed before me. Huge mansions with acres of land and a fleet of Bentleys and Porsches on the gravel drive. Yes, it was safe to say I'd moved a few times since then.

It turned out I'd last been to the hospital twenty-seven years earlier, when I was seven years old. As I stood leaning on the reception desk, I had a flashback of falling over on bonfire night. I cut my head and needed seven stitches above my right eye. I still had the scar to prove it, and I remembered how it hurt like mad and I had tried hard not to cry with pain. Now here I was aged 34, in pain again but this time unable to stop the tears rolling down my face.

Victoria sat with me patiently, phoned my parents and tried to keep me chatting and awake. Victoria is a great girl. She sings in a band called Red Addiction and had a gig later that night. She talked about her music and told me how her little daughter Livia always played so beautifully with Lina. I remember she said how great it was that I was living back in Swansea, living close to so many friends and family. 'Thank God for that,' I thought.

I was aware of people staring at me, but I couldn't care less. I've no idea if they recognised me or were just thinking, 'What's up with that poor bastard?' We sat in A & E for about two hours, waiting to be seen. My head was bursting and my eyes were closing. At one point I staggered to the toilets and threw up. What I saw terrified me, and I started shouting while I was still vomiting. It was that dark, watery liquid I'd vomited up at home earlier. I started cursing and screaming at it. What the hell was it? It didn't look like normal sick. It was something very unfamiliar and sinister-looking, and that freaked me out. I washed it down the sink. It scared me just to look at it. 'Get away from me!' I yelled. 'Go on, get away!'

When I sat back down on the plastic chair in the waiting room, I could hardly hold my head up. I curled myself up, cradled my head in my hands and willed myself to keep my eyes open. It was no use. The pain was so sharp it felt like physical blows raining down on my head. I started moaning and wailing. My eyes were like wafer-thin slits in my face. The pain was literally blinding me. I have a vague memory of retching again and again and throwing up more of that putrid liquid. It felt like it came from the darkest corners of my lungs and stomach, and I had no control over it. My dad turned up at the hospital. 'I heard you before I saw you,' he said. I was making a desperate, sickening sound as I puked my guts up, or whatever the hell it was I was puking up.

I can't tell you what happened next. My eyes finally gave up. The thin slits closed over completely and everything went black. I have virtually no memory of the next four or five weeks.

CHAPTER SEVEN

'Am I gonna live, doctor?'

SARAH

I stood on our sloping driveway for a few moments and watched John and Victoria drive off down the road. The warm afternoon sun wrapped itself across the back of my shoulders, but I gave a little shiver. Something was wrong. Had I misjudged John's headaches? Had the 'hangover' from Dublin been a complete red herring? I shuddered when I remembered what I'd said jokingly to my sister Frances on the phone one day that week. 'That'll teach him!' I had mockingly cursed. I scolded myself now. 'Don't be silly,' a voice said in my head. 'Pull yourself together. Go in and get Lina. Go to the hospital and find out what's what.'

Lina did an excited dance across the carpet when I saw her. 'She's been a little angel,' Louise told me brightly. 'No trouble at all.' I went through the motions of giving Lina some fish and mashed potato for her tea and chatting to her as she pointed excitedly at CBeebies on the telly, but my nerves were jangling. I wanted to see John.

'Let's go see Daddy!' I smiled.

'Da-da, da-da. Want Daddy!' Lina beamed, throwing her arms up high for me to pick her up and carry her to the car. As I strapped her into her car seat I thought about her birth. That was the last time I had been in the Singleton Hospital. I shuddered again.

My pregnancy had been perfect. I felt fantastic, and I was thrilled I was expecting a little girl. It's what John and I had hoped for. I was completely chilled out even in the last, uncomfortable months, and couldn't wait for the birth. We all expected the delivery to be normal, but Lina had other ideas. At the last minute she tried to come out forehead and face first, which made the delivery anything but normal. The technical term is 'brow presentation'. The midwife blanched, John went as white as a sheet and I was crying with pain and fear. It was dangerous for both of us, but it was too late to stop her. The words 'emergency Caesarean' rang out. I was terrified. This wasn't what I had planned at all. When Lina's wee body was finally lifted from me, her face was all grazed and bloodied and she made no sound. I will never forget the silence. The room was in chaos, with doctors and nurses and midwives rushing around, wheeling equipment, snatching Lina away from me, checking her eyes and heartbeat and her fingers and toes. It was pandemonium, but it was silent.

My stomach churned as I walked back through the doors of the Singleton and headed to A & E. I clutched Lina tightly to my chest. I didn't want either of us to see John in pain, and in my mind's eye I imagined him sitting quietly with Victoria, perhaps resting his eyes and waiting patiently for his turn to be seen. I stopped in my tracks in the corridor when I realised the man being pushed towards me in a wheelchair was John. He was crumpled over in the chair, his head lolling forward, and he looked completely delirious, moaning in pain and barely conscious. 'John!' I called out. 'Oh my God! Can somebody please tell me what's going on?'

I didn't want to frighten Lina, so I kept myself calm, found a doctor and asked him for an update. He told me they were going to take some blood and do an assessment on John, and he was being put in a ward. He added that John might have some kind of a virus, which would explain the sickness and headaches, and said that he was being booked in for a brain scan the next day to try to get to the root of the headaches. 'Brain scan?' I repeated. I was flabbergasted. It sounded scary, and I was confused.

I had no idea John had already been diagnosed with testicular cancer the day before. He hadn't got round to telling me, and nothing was making sense. I clung onto the word 'virus'. It seemed the most logical explanation. After all, I'd seen him walking out of our front door a couple of hours earlier. He couldn't be that bad.

I found John on Ward Two. He was lying in a sparse but neat little bay with its own television, but it was switched off and he seemed quite oblivious to his surroundings. He had the sheets pulled round his face and was trying to sleep, but he was really restless and clearly in a lot of pain.

'We'll make him as comfortable as we can,' a friendly male nurse reassured me. John's dad, Cyril, had been out to Sainsbury's with Victoria to buy some fresh fruit. They looked shattered when they walked in but tried to act as normal as possible, arranging the grapes and tangerines in a bowl and making a fuss of Lina. We talked about John's mum, Diana. She was due to go on a cruise the next day with her friend Carole. It was leaving from Belgium, and she had told Cyril she had a 'bad feeling' about John's headaches and thought she should cancel. 'I've told her to go,' Cyril said. Even John opened his eyes at one stage and muttered that his mum should go, and we all nodded in agreement. I think it made us all feel better, convincing ourselves that John's condition would soon improve.

I left John sleeping and eventually went home feeling very uneasy. The house felt huge and empty with just Lina and me there. We have seven television screens hanging off various walls in the house, and when John is at home there's invariably a football match, golf tournament or rugby game blaring out of one or two of them. I often left him to it and tuned into *EastEnders* or *Coronation Street* in another room, but I'd grin to myself whenever I heard him cheering on players or berating the referee. I liked his noise and bustle. I liked just having him under the same roof as me. I missed him.

Once Lina was settled in her cot, I didn't know really what to do with myself. I phoned my mum in Fort William. 'You might need to give me a hand with Lina,' I found myself saying. 'I think John needs me more than she does right now.' I called my sister Frances, too. She's a nurse, and I value her advice and opinion very highly. She readily agreed to

127

help out. 'You know how much my kids like to see Lina,' she said. 'She'll have a ball up here. Me and Mum will fix it. You concentrate on John.' When I put the phone down I had mixed feelings. I felt very grateful that my family had swung into action so willingly, but I had a horrible pang of fear too. Having Lina whisked away to Scotland was an acknowledgement of the seriousness of the situation.

I didn't sleep well. I thought of the nights I had moaned at John for snoring and breathing too heavily. It seemed so petty now. I'd have given anything to have him back in our bed, noise or no noise. I thought about how bad his breathing had sounded recently, and it scared me. I think the only thing that made me finally drop off was thinking about the new baby. I knew I had to look after myself in those early stages of pregnancy. I was only a month down the line. It was a crucial time, and I promised myself I would eat and sleep and rest as best I could.

VICTORIA'S DIARY

Saturday, 11 July 2009

I decided to write this diary for John to look back at everything he has been through once he has made a full recovery. As John is in and out of sleep, I thought there would be times he wouldn't be able to remember. This is for John to know exactly what he has been through and the treatment he has received. I'd like John to know about the messages of support he is receiving from across the country. Hearing John's news has really shaken everybody up. Finally, I hope this will be a great testament to just how much of a fighter John really is.

SARAH

When I arrived at the hospital on Saturday, John was just about to go for his brain scan. He was lying down and was on a drip for pain relief, but he still looked to be in agony. I kissed his cheek and stroked his arm, but he was barely able to acknowledge me. His eyes were half closed and his face was etched with pain. He looked helpless, and I felt helpless too. I sat with Victoria while John was wheeled off for the scan. Victoria told me that earlier that morning John had tried to eat a few bits of fruit but couldn't keep anything down. He threw up that awful murky liquid again.

By now I think I'd stopped trying to convince myself the situation would somehow miraculously improve. John had clearly got worse overnight, and even being drip-fed painkillers wasn't relieving him at all. I was starting to feel impatient and anxious. John had been in hospital for almost 24 hours now, yet we were none the wiser about his condition and he was enduring worse pain than ever. I didn't have a clue how the hospital worked in terms of scans and tests, and I worried that things were moving slower than normal because it was a weekend. The consultant, Dr Harris, came in to see me and said ominously: 'We need to have a chat.' I nodded and agreed to meet him at 6.30 p.m., along with Cyril. The waiting was unbearable. When John came back from his scan I just sat there with Cyril for what seemed like hours, watching John grimace through his pain. I didn't know what to say to cheer him up. He looked broken.

My heart leapt when Dr Harris eventually reappeared with the scan results. I scoured his face for news. He looked grave as he gestured for me and Cyril to step outside. We sprang up and walked out onto the ward. I was practically holding my breath I was so desperate for news. 'Actually,' said Dr Harris thoughtfully. 'Let's go back inside and tell you what's happened in front of John. No doubt he will be concerned with us not being in the room.'

My heart was pounding now, and Cyril looked petrified. Dr Harris cleared his throat and I gripped the metal at the foot of John's bed. 'We have done the brain scan and it's not entirely normal.'

I felt the blood drain from my legs and thought I was going to collapse. Dr Harris's words swam around my head, making me feel dizzy. He talked about the lump in John's testicle. I heard him say 'testicular cancer'. And finally I heard him say: 'I'm afraid the testicular cancer has spread to his brain.'

There was a moment of silence, then John's voice cut through the air. 'Am I gonna live, doctor?' I felt so bad just looking at him. He was grey and he looked panic-stricken.

'It's uncertain what is going to happen,' said Dr Harris. 'We will have to do further tests.' He added something along the lines of 'you've got more than half a chance'.

I sat in silence for a few moments, struggling to take in the enormity of what I'd heard. This was the first I knew of John's testicular cancer. To find out your partner has cancer is bad enough, but I was reeling from three sets of bad news all at once. John had testicular cancer. It had spread to his brain. And the doctor hadn't said 'yes' when John asked if he was going to survive.

> My dad and Sarah were naturally in shock and began the phone calls to close family. 6.30 p.m. was the longest minute coming ever. Time froze. I was waiting for a call from my daddy and hoping it was good news. When I answered the phone he said, 'Bad news, Vic,' and then started crying. I knew straight away; he needn't tell me any more. I was sitting outside my bandmate Louise's house, as we had a gig. She drove and I was just speechless and upset, but at least now we knew what the pains were. Daddy phoned Mammy around 7.30 p.m. He couldn't possibly keep it from her; she'd never forgive him. John wasn't doing very well. He was struggling to breathe and sleep and was also upset on hearing the news. Big James said he had a great chance and we all needed to remain positive.

SARAH

I was in a terrible state on Sunday. I had hardly slept a wink and I remember being first to arrive at the hospital. John had been moved to Ward Eleven the night before. I did a depressing double take when I followed the signs to oncology. John was on a cancer ward. He was officially a cancer patient. I couldn't take it in at all. I was relieved to see him sitting up in bed when I arrived, but when he spoke he wasn't himself at all. To this day he can barely remember a thing about his first four or five weeks in hospital, even the times when he was conscious and talking. He seemed spaced out and disorientated.

John's older sister Hayley arrived, followed by John's old friend Colin Payne, his cousin Mark Hartson, who is also one of John's closest friends, plus Cyril, who had helped make arrangements for John's mum, Diana, to travel home from her cruise.

The situation felt quite surreal. Normally this crowd of people would only gather together at a family party, but here we all were at the hospital. The lads cracked jokes and chatted about old times. Colin ran the local club, where John had worked as a glass collector when he was a teenager. They've been mates for ever, and Colin was doing daft impressions, just as if the pair of them were sitting having a pint. Mark put on a good show too. He's grown up with John and now lives three doors away from us. They're as thick as thieves and, somehow, John found the strength to join in the lads' banter. I was grateful for the distraction. 'Paul Glover's coming down from Nottingham,' John chimed in at one stage. Paul is another great old friend. 'Glovers can't miss out on nothing,' John joked. 'He has to be in on all the action.'

I looked at John and felt so proud. He was at such a low ebb, propped up in bed half naked, hooked up to a painkilling drip, but he was still making an effort to entertain his friends. It was typical of him. I was also grateful he had such close friends who cared so deeply for him. They seemed to have perked him up, and when I heard that more were on the way I was pleased for John. He was still using his phone from time to time, and he told me his close friends Tommy, Wayne, Lee and Karl were all on their way too.

Despite the bravado and banter, I could tell John was still in a lot of pain. He looked like he was trying not to move his head too much, and he kept squinting, as if the pain was pressing behind his eyes. 'Is there nothing else you can do to relieve his pain?' I asked the nurse quietly. She checked John's drip. He was already on a high dose of morphine for pain relief and had been prescribed 15 steroid tablets a day to shrink the tumours in his brain. 'We're doing the best we can,' she said apologetically. It was stressful not knowing what would happen next, but nobody seemed to be telling us anything.

131

As the hours ticked by, I started to worry about John's mental state. At one point he spoke to Rebeca and Joni on his mobile phone, which put a smile on his face. But then he started crying and fretting. I think the medication was getting to him, and he seemed confused and disorientated. He asked if the children could come in and see him. None of us had any experience of how to deal with a patient in John's condition, and at first we naturally tried to grant all of his wishes. If he wanted to see the children, then of course he should. I'd taken Lina in to see him very briefly and she seemed to perk him up, but it was easy with Lina. She was only a baby. She didn't bat an eyelid about Daddy being in a strange bed with tubes sticking out of him.

I didn't argue, though. As I said, I'm no expert. None of us were. The children visited at lunchtime, and John's face immediately brightened. He looked so pleased to see them and he managed to chat away quite coherently.

When they left, John had tears running down his face and started saying loudly: 'Make sure my kids are OK. If anything happens to me, make sure my kids are OK.' It was unbearably sad. John's kids are his world. He absolutely adores all of them. To look at him lying there, fearing leaving them behind, was devastating.

Dr Gianfilippo Bertelli, the consultant oncologist at Singleton, came to see John. He told John this was treatable and curable. In most cases of testicular cancer there is a 95 per cent success rate. However, because John's had spread there was an 80 per cent success rate. We all felt quite positive on hearing this news. Also we were informed by other staff how fantastic Dr Bertelli was and how lucky they were to have him at the hospital. Dr Bertelli was Italian and very smart and professional.

Mam caught a series of shuttle buses, trains and two flights, from Brussels to Edinburgh and on to Cardiff. Big James collected her from the airport and brought her straight to the hospital. It was 11 p.m. by the time she arrived. John was pleased to see her but got emotional, and he was in terrible pain. We were all asking for more pain relief and discussing amongst ourselves how surely more could be done to get him out of pain, as nothing the doctors and nurses were giving him seemed to be working or even making things slightly better – in fact, he was getting worse.

SARAH

I was nervous about John's mum arriving. I'd seen how emotional he became when he had his loved ones around him, and I feared he might break down completely.

When she finally walked down the corridor, she had been travelling for a full 15 hours. Diana is normally bright and breezy, but she looked absolutely dreadful. She had driven herself mad on the journey, imagining all kinds. And when she emerged from John's room after finally seeing him, she looked even worse.

'Poor John,' she said, tears streaming down her face. 'I can't believe that is my John lying there.' Diana sat in the waiting room and sobbed. She looked exhausted and petrified, and my heart went out to her.

Driving home alone, I imagined what it must have felt like for Diana, not being there for all those hours. I wanted to stay by John's side and never leave him, but I knew I had to get home to Lina. Everybody had been so good. Friends and neighbours had rallied round to help care for her while I was at the hospital, but Lina needed me too.

She was fast asleep when I got home, and I went straight to bed. My body was aching all over and I forced myself to think of our new baby. I was in such an early stage of pregnancy that I knew I had to sleep and take care of myself. I had to be strong while John was so weak. I shut my eyes and willed myself to sleep, pushing dark thoughts out of my head. They weren't going to help anyone. I was not going to be frightened by them. I was going to fight, just as John had to fight. Tomorrow he was having a blast of radiotherapy to shrink the tumours in his brain. Then he was having a CAT scan to search his whole body for cancer. It was going to be a very tough day.

Monday, 13 July

Sarah dropped Lina off to me at 8.30 a.m. I took her to nursery with my Livia. Livia loved showing off her baby cousin to her friends, and Lina was in her element.

John received his first radiotherapy session and he seemed to cope fine with it. It only lasts a few minutes, but it's very intense, just like blasting the head to reduce the tumours. We were all pleased that some sort of treatment was taking place.

SARAH

I felt impatient when I arrived at the hospital. I walked directly to Ward Eleven as if I'd trodden the path a million times already, even though John had only been in there since Saturday. The weekend had felt like it lasted an eternity. We'd had John's diagnosis, but nothing else seemed to happen. It was as if we had been just waiting around for Monday morning, waiting for more tests and more results. All I wanted was for treatment to begin. I had these horrible images in my mind of the tumours growing and multiplying, and I just wanted them to stop. I just wanted him to be blasted with radiotherapy and chemotherapy and whatever else it took to kill the cancer fast, before it did any more damage. 'You're making progress now, John,' I told him as he was wheeled off for his radiotherapy. 'Your treatment is starting. The radiotherapy will help you get better.'

The nurse had told me he had had a tough night, struggling to breathe. 'Can you hear me, John? Squeeze my hand if you can,' I said. He was dosed up to the eyeballs with painkillers, but he gave me the weakest squeeze. I kissed the top of his head as he disappeared into the radiotherapy unit, but he didn't respond.

As I arrived in the ward and went into John's room, he didn't look well and was just about to go for his CAT scan. My dad and I walked down with John to the area of the hospital where they take place, and while he had it we had a little cry. My dad was finding it difficult to see John in so much pain and feeling very uncomfortable. On top of that my dad had a bit of a heart-to-heart with John before he went down, and he told John: 'You're a strong boy, you've got so much to live for.'

While John was in having the scan, a nurse called me and my dad aside and said the press were outside wanting to film John going back to the ward. At this point we were assured there would be no filming and my dad also went outside to ask them to respect the family's wishes and not film.

The porters helped shield John's trolley on his return to the ward and my dad pulled the sheet over his head, just in case they were filming. They didn't film John, but Dr Bertelli was filmed reading out a statement, and all the ward and admin managers were informed of the press situation and told not to let them into the wards.

John was front page on the *Scottish Sun* that day and news had spread to other newspapers and TV news from there.

John returned to Ward Eleven and was trying to rest, but he found it impossible. He couldn't get comfortable, his breathing was getting worse and he was getting agitated. When he was coming round and whenever his painkillers were wearing off, John would kind of wake up in shock and try to pull the tubes and wires out of himself.

Sarah

It was terrible watching John suffer. By late evening most of his visitors had left, and for a little while I was sitting alone with John. He'd been put on a high dose of the steroid dexamethasone as soon as the cancer in his brain was discovered, he had an oxygen mask to help his breathing and he had been put on a catheter. He looked gravely ill.

My mind went into overdrive whenever I was alone. I tossed around all the facts I knew, trying to make sense of them, trying to weigh up the possibilities and trying to convince myself everything was going to be all right and John would pull through.

I'd been told that the cancer markers in John's blood measured 191,000. This was one of the many details to emerge about John's condition after his initial blood tests, but it took a few days for me to really allow the seriousness of this detail to sink in. The oncologist told me that in a healthy person the number is generally in single figures. Sitting beside John's bed, seeing him looking so desperately ill, I was having trouble putting a positive spin on those numbers. I heard the words 'riddled' and 'uncontrollable' bouncing around my head, but I tried my best to push them away.

'When the chemo kicks in they can drop quite rapidly at first, then the drop will normally plateau.' Someone had said that too, and that's the phrase I pulled to the front of my mind as I watched over John that night.

'I should warn you that John may experience what we call "steroid psychosis",' one of the nurses mentioned when she came in to check on John. She had heard me chatting to John, trying to get him to respond, and I think she was worried about what his response might be. 'What I mean is, he may hallucinate and say peculiar things. Don't be alarmed. It is just the drugs.'

'OK, I understand.'

Almost as soon as the nurse left the room, John took his hand out of mine and slowly pulled away his oxygen mask. All his movements were very slow and gentle, and for a moment I imagined he was going to tell me he loved me, like cancer patients do in films.

But instead John snarled: 'I know all about it, Sarah.' His voice was deep and rasping. He didn't even sound like my John, and I jumped up in alarm. 'I know all about your affair with that male nurse! Don't try to deny it! I know, babe! I know!'

It took my breath away, and I really didn't know how to respond. 'Don't shout, John,' I said, trying to calm him down. 'It's just the drugs. I'm not cheating on you, John. I would never do that. I love you, John.'

'Where's my dad?' he growled. 'Is he out on the piss again? Is he? Is he? I've told him not to get pissed. How could he while I'm lying here?'

I didn't know what to say. John was getting himself in a terrible state and I didn't have a clue how to handle him. 'John, there is no bar here.

Your dad is in the visitor's room. He's been here round the clock, keeping an eye on you and helping you get better.

'Why don't you just try to relax,' I said gently. 'I'll get the nurse to fix your oxygen . . .' Before I finished my sentence, John ripped off his sheets and leapt out of bed, angrily pulling every tube out of his body.

'I'm getting out of here!' he hissed. 'Get out of my way! You can't stop me!' He was dressed in boxer shorts and looked like the Incredible Hulk, snarling and cursing as he threw his pipes and drips aside and tried to make a desperate lurch for the door.

'John, no!' I cried, trying to restrain him. John's parents and a nurse heard the commotion and all ran in to help me, but it was too late. John was flailing around unsteadily on his feet, but he was too heavy for any of us to hold.

One of the nurses tried to block him, but he barged on and nearly put her through the wall. The next moment his strength seemed to disappear. His feet went from under him, and he fell face first into a metal trolley. The thud ended the commotion, and he finally allowed a nurse to settle him back in bed, treat the shiner that started to swell on his eye and re-plug his tubes. We all sat in horrified silence. I felt sick to my stomach. John was breathing very heavily now and was complaining of pains in his chest.

'I can't cough,' he said. 'I've got something stuck in my throat.' I didn't know whether he was imagining things again. 'I'm going home with you, Sarah,' he shouted. 'I'm getting out of here!' We all pleaded with him to stay put and not pull out his tubes again, but it was no use. He suddenly sat bolt upright, ripped them off all over again and sat up on all fours on the bed.

'John, please lie back down. Please don't get off the bed. You're not even meant to sit up . . .'

I went to hold his arms, but he pushed me away. Even in his weakened state John was strong, and he launched his huge bulk towards the door and made his escape. Before we could stop him he was lolloping down the corridor, drips and wires swinging off him as he shouted loudly, 'I'm getting out of here. Come on, Sarah, we're going home!'

I looked at the ruffled sheet left behind on his bed and the machines frantically bleeping all around. It was like a ludicrous scene from a bad medical drama.

Eventually it was Cyril who got a grip on him and helped guide him back to bed, but not without a struggle. 'Don't tell me what to do – you're drunk,' he accused his dad loudly. 'You've had too much to drink at the bar!'

'I think we need to move wards,' a nurse said eventually. 'We think he will be better off in the coronary care unit, where we can keep a closer eye on him.' I felt useless. I wanted to help, but I was just beholden to whatever the medical staff told me. I didn't understand why coronary care would be a better place and I worried that the nurses just wanted to move him because they couldn't cope with him. He didn't have anything wrong with his heart, did he? It felt like we'd taken a step backwards, having to move to a higher-dependency ward, and I had a horrible feeling that things were going to get a lot worse before they got better.

I met my parents outside the coronary care unit and they looked exhausted, not to mention worried. Inside, John opened his eyes to see me, but he really wasn't with it. James was there, too. We got John to drink and changed his pillows and put his light and fan on and off, trying to get him comfortable, but nothing was working. John's breathing was awful. We couldn't work out why his chest was so bad. He couldn't seem to cough. We kept telling him to lie back and breathe and turn on his side if it was more comfortable for him. Nothing was working. It was really upsetting. We felt helpless. John jumped out of bed again and James and I tried to restrain him, but he was telling us we were holding him against his own will. He was just standing there trying to maintain his balance. We managed to get him back in the bed, but then he wouldn't lie down. He was telling the nurse to 'get off', saying, 'Who do you think you are, touching my arm like that?' I pulled the nurse to one side after John had calmed down a little to tell her he wasn't usually like this. She was fine and said they were used to it. John tried to sleep, but his snoring was so bad that within 30 seconds he woke himself up. Then he stood by the side of the bed and started hallucinating. He thought he was in the casino playing dice, then chips. 'Come on, boy,' he said to James, pretending to shake the dice. We tried to get him to sit down, but he was having none of it. His eyes were shut, but he was talking so fast. He'd sit down then get up, then lay down. Then he started shouting: 'Football, five-a-side – come on kids, we're off!' I started getting upset. I felt so hopeless.

SARAH

Eventually John fell into a relatively peaceful sleep, and Cyril and I sat together in a sort of stunned silence, keeping watch over him. Cyril is a big, proud man, just like John, and he was doing a magnificent job in the circumstances. He gave regular updates to the visitors, he kept the press informed and I even heard him chatting away to the nurses in the lifts and corridors, making them laugh and lightening the atmosphere. Diana was extremely emotional, and he calmed her down too and tried to reassure her as much as he could. Most importantly, Cyril spent a lot of time saying reassuring things to John. 'It's going well, son. You're being well cared for. You're in the right place. When you get out of here, we'll have a game of darts and a few pints together. Don't you worry.'

We lost track of time. The bleeps of the machines quickly became a familiar background noise. The chemical smells of the cleaning fluids and drugs were second nature. Nothing seemed to matter except the sound of John's breathing. When it was stable, I felt more relaxed.

'Sarah, you go and get some rest,' Cyril said. 'I'll keep watch over him. You need to look after that little grandchild of mine you're carrying.'

I felt better knowing Cyril was staying and John was not alone. I stood up slowly, my bones creaking from having sat for so long, and suddenly John sat bolt upright too.

'Don't let them do it, Dad!' he shouted. 'I know they've measured me up. I know what they are planning. I've seen the machines. Don't let them! Please, don't let them, Daddy!'

Cyril told him firmly and calmly there was nothing at all to worry about. 'I am here,' he said. 'Don't worry, John. I am keeping an eye on you. Nobody is going to hurt you.'

'No, Dad, you don't understand!' John ranted. He was screaming loudly now, and Cyril was standing over him, ready to grab him if he tried to leap off the bed.

'What don't I understand, John?'

'They are going to cut off my arms and legs, Daddy. They are going to amputate my arms and legs. Whatever you do, don't let them do that. Please.'

It was a heart-stopping moment. I felt so desperately sorry for John. He was so confused and scared, just like a little boy.

'Oh my God,' I cried. 'Cyril, this is horrific.'

Thankfully John fell silent and allowed Cyril to help him back onto his pillow. I stroked his forehead. The moment was gone, and John shut his eyes and started breathing deeply, if erratically.

Chapter Eight

'Please don't go'

Tuesday, 14 July

In the morning, John still wasn't doing very well. He was kind of in and out of consciousness, his headaches were still there and he was on every drug under the sun – morphine, steroids and temazepam. When Mum spoke to the doctors and nurses, she said he should be moved from coronary care to intensive care because he'd have one-to-one care there, and they agreed. As a family, we felt a little bit like the nurses were intimidated by John and his size and the way he was pulling all the pipes out and taking these funny turns and wanting to go home. Once John was settled into intensive care, we were all pleased. We were introduced to the consultant, Paul, who explained the way ITU works, with visitors kept low.

At around 1 p.m., Dr Bertelli came to visit us to give us the results of the CAT scan. He called us into a private room. Our hearts were in our throats, as these were the results we'd all been waiting for. You could see the worry in Dr Bertelli's face, and we all waited in anticipation. He couldn't say it quick enough. 'I'm afraid John's cancer has spread to his lungs and the lymphs around the abdomen.' He went into detail to say there was still a lot of hope, and now that he had been moved to the intensive care unit they would be able to keep more of an eye on him. We were all gutted to hear that it had spread, but we did half expect to hear it, as we were fairly realistic and knew that the cancer was bound to have spread elsewhere between the testicle and the brain. We all bombarded Dr Bertelli with questions about future treatment. He said they were going to give him an immediate dose of radiotherapy, a one-off session, to try to kick-start the treatment to the lungs and lower abdomen, but at this point John wasn't well enough to have chemotherapy, as they suspected pneumonia had set in. We asked the fatal question: 'What are his chances?', and he replied: '50–50'. He also said, 'I'd be lying if I told you I wasn't a worried man.' Well, our hearts sank. Things were just going from bad to worse. We were all concerned that without the chemo the tumours would grow, but we were told they had to take things one step at a time.

SARAH

My sister Frances and my mum arrived from Scotland to look after Lina. I was dreading seeing them, because I knew I wouldn't be able to hold it together in front of them the way I could with other people. They met me at the hospital, and I relayed the news from Dr Bertelli through a stream of tears that flowed faster with every word. It didn't seem real. Normally we chatted about the kids, holidays, clothes, washing machines, films, schools – anything under the sun but this. It was so alien. 'Can we pop in and see him for a wee minute?' Frances asked. I nodded quietly. I love Frances to pieces. She is my only sibling and we're very close. I've always trusted her judgement, and as she's a nurse I found myself hanging on her every word. I watched her intently as she edged into John's room. My mum shuffled in beside her. She is a very stoical person, but neither she nor Frances could hide their reaction on seeing John lying there. They visibly blanched.

John had an oxygen mask over his face and drips attached all over the place feeding him morphine, steroids and the tranquilliser temazepam. His eyes were rolling round his head, but he suddenly focused on Frances and his face crumpled. Tears began streaming down his cheeks. John knows how close I am to Frances, and I wondered if he was crying with relief and gratitude that she was there to help me, while he was so helpless.

My mum and sister both looked distraught, and another thought darted across my head. Did John think this was his last farewell to my family? Is that what Frances and my mum thought too? 'My God, it doesn't look good, Sarah,' Frances said when we left the room. My heart tightened. I felt a cold fear trickle through my veins.

Frances had voiced what I already knew to be true deep inside, but hearing her words bouncing off the bare walls in the hospital corridor sharpened my focus and stripped away any doubt. There was no way you could dress this up. John was in a very bad state, and for the first time I really acknowledged that I could lose him.

Later, when I was holding Lina, I saw John in her eyes, and it gave me strength and hope. 'Your daddy will make it,' I told her. 'He's young and strong and he'll fight like a lion,' I thought. 'He has every chance of pulling through. No way is this a farewell.'

When I waved my mum and sister off with Lina, I felt bereft. It was her first birthday that day. I'd barely given it a thought and hadn't even bought her a present, let alone baked the pink cake I'd planned for her party tea. 'Happy Birthday from Mummy and Daddy,' I said as I kissed her on the cheek and waved goodbye. I was aware I was using that sing-songy voice parents do when they're trying to pretend everything is normal when it's anything but. 'See you soon. Have fun with your cousins, Lina!'

I wanted our family back to normal, but I sensed I had a long wait. I'd packed two weeks' worth of clothes and nappies for Lina, but surely she wouldn't need to be away for that long? The voice of reason that was standing up for itself in my head told me this was simply the sensible thing to do, rather than an indicator of how ill John was. Hospitals are no place for babies. They don't understand what is happening, and children always make emotional situations more highly charged. Every time I had looked at Lina in the last few days, it felt like I had another emotional dart stabbing my heart. Her image stirred up a maelstrom of love and hope and fear. It was very hard to cope with, and I had no doubt she was better off in Scotland so I could focus on John's recovery.

Before we said goodbye, Frances took me to one side and said she was concerned about the number of visitors John had received. We had already been told he had suspected pneumonia, which he must have picked up in his first few days in hospital. Frances explained how serious this was. It would not only set back his cancer treatment, which was clearly extremely bad news; in his weakened state, it could actually kill him.

A nurse had explained to me that John was meant to have nil by mouth, but well-meaning visitors had brought in grapes and offered him sips of water. As John wasn't breathing or swallowing properly, a piece of food had probably travelled to his lungs and got stuck there, growing bacteria and causing the infection that led to pneumonia.

Frances said she was concerned about John catching other infections, too. I hadn't even thought about that. I'd lost count of the number of relatives and friends who had gathered in the last four days. Their reaction was extremely touching. Some had travelled miles and abandoned their jobs just to pop in for a few minutes or sit in the waiting room.

The hospital had moved them into a bigger visitors' room because there were so many of them. Someone joked that they'd have to call it the 'Hartson Lounge' and pin up some of John's football shirts and get him to do an official opening when he was better. It was all good morale-boosting talk, but now it didn't seem so funny. It was clearly time to limit the number of visitors going to his bedside.

Bec and Joni had been nagging to see John, and the intensive care consultant, Paul, agreed that Hayley could take them in. Unfortunately Hayley got really upset, which upset John and the children, and they all started to have a good cry. The consultant said it was too distressing for John and it wasn't to happen again. Every time he saw people, he was getting really emotional. He was trying to talk but was linked up to so many tubes and machines it was difficult. Plus, all the different concoctions of drugs he was on were making him really confused.

SARAH

Later that afternoon I sat alone with John, holding his hand. Paul, the intensive care doctor, came in and told me he was going off shift. 'Is there anything you want to ask before I go?' he asked. I'd got used to the constant beeping around John and I glanced at the machines. To my untrained eye, everything appeared fine. John's heart rate and oxygen levels were stable.

'No, I don't think . . .' As I spoke, I could hear John's breathing getting heavier and heavier. Suddenly he was gasping for air inside his oxygen mask, making a desperate 'yhurghh, yhuuurghh' noise. My eyes darted to the oxygen machine plugged up beside his bed and I saw the numbers start to plummet. Sixty, fifty-two, forty . . . I didn't understand what they meant; I just knew they shouldn't be dropping so quickly. Panic rising in my voice, I shouted out, 'Paul, what's happening?' Paul was shouting too, but all I could see were his lips moving. An emergency alarm was ringing out from the oxygen machine, drowning out every other sound. In the blink of an eye, the room was spilling over with stony-faced doctors and nurses all fastening up their white aprons as they dashed to John's bedside with tubes and drips and equipment. Fear flooded my body. Nobody spoke a word. It felt like I was in the middle of utter pandemonium, but it was silent pandemonium. It reminded me of the eerie chaos in the long minutes after Lina's traumatic birth. I could see white coats dashing everywhere, trolleys being wheeled in, machines flashing and tubes and wires being plugged frantically into John. It was like watching a silent movie, and the silence scared me. Suddenly an awful realisation hit me. I realised the sound of John's desperate breathing had gone too. That's why my whole world had gone quiet. 'Oh my God, no!' I cried. 'He's stopped breathing!' I stopped one of the male nurses in his tracks. 'Tell me he's OK? Tell me he's going to be OK? He looked at the floor, unable to make eye contact with me, then scuttled into the store cupboard. The digital numbers on John's oxygen machine had disappeared completely now and it was making that flat, lifeless beeping sound I'd only ever heard when someone died on *Casualty*. I ran outside, shouting for Cyril and Diana.

145

'He's stopped breathing!' I sobbed. Their faces were ashen. Dr Bertelli was in with John now, and all we could do was wait anxiously for news. None of us spoke. What could you say?

When Dr Bertelli finally called us in, he looked very serious. I was holding my breath in fear as he spoke. 'We are going to have to perform an emergency brain operation,' he said. My heart thumped.

I listened intently as Dr Bertelli explained that the large tumour at the top of John's spine was stopping the blood draining away as it normally should. The resulting pressure was so great it was pressing on the brain stem: the part of John's brain that told him to breathe. This might have been a result of the radiotherapy triggering an initial swelling in the tumour as it worked to shrink it, which is a normal response.

They would have to drill into John's skull and insert a drain in the back of his head to draw off excess fluid, relieve the pressure and help him breathe again. In the meantime, they would replace John's oxygen mask with a ventilator pipe inserted down his throat to force him to breathe artificially.

It was a lot to take in. 'Will I lose him?' was all I said. I could hardly believe the words had come out of my mouth.

'The issue now is saving John's life,' Dr Bertelli said gravely. 'The cancer treatment comes second.' I started gasping for air. My lungs felt crushed and I couldn't get any air into them at all, however hard I tried. I thought I was going to faint. Cyril broke down too. I was clinging onto John's metal bedstead to stop myself falling down.

'John, please don't go,' Cyril cried. 'Don't leave us, John. Please don't go.' His legs buckled too. Diana clutched his arm. She was sobbing hysterically. It was painful just to look at them suffering so much distress.

All the bad news crashed about in my head. In just a few days, John's diagnosis had gone from a bad headache to a suspected virus and then testicular cancer that wasn't just in his testicle, but his brain and lungs, too. I felt sick and dizzy. I thought it couldn't get much worse, and now this. Now he needed an emergency brain operation to save his life.

Paul came into the waiting room to tell us that John had stopped breathing. He explained that the pressure on his head and the pneumonia had probably got too much for John to deal with, but he'd booked him in for a scan to see exactly what was going on and then they would think about a plan of action. The waiting room was now packed and the wait for the scan, even though it was only about 20 minutes, felt like hours.

John's friends Wayne and Tommy arrived, and Paul Glover drove back from Nottingham and told work he would not be returning until John was well. Karl and Mark had been there more or less since Sunday.

Paul, the consultant, called us all into the bigger waiting room (because there were so many of us) and again delivered bad news. John had to travel to Morriston Hospital immediately to have emergency surgery to relieve the fluid on his brain, as that was probably the reason he had stopped breathing. He told us that throughout the day the neurosurgeons at Morriston had been aware of John and were available to operate if need be.

I went out into the corridor to make a few phone calls and so did others. We were all petrified.

I decided to nip down to see John in ITU before he travelled to Morriston. My nephew, Baby James, was with me. When we entered the unit, my dad was standing at the side of John's bed and he was crying terrible. I've never seen someone so upset in my whole life. This really shook up Baby James and me. Baby James started having a panic attack. He couldn't get his breath and was almost fainting. The doctors came with some paper bags and I slowly started walking Baby James back to the waiting room, and Karl looked after him from there. I went back down to see John, and it was my turn to lose it a bit. I just got so upset seeing John and seeing the effect it was having on my parents.

I prayed and prayed and asked everyone to pray. I had a lot of faith in Mamgu, in ensuring she would make sure John stayed with us. I felt she was watching over us and I was sure it wasn't his time to go.

SARAH

After days and days of feeling stuck in slow motion, suddenly everything was happening at a rate of knots. 'Every hour is critical now,' Paul, the consultant, told me. John was whisked away for a brain scan and was also given an emergency dose of chemotherapy, administered via a drip. Paul explained that it was vital to get to the Morriston quickly because it had a specialist neurosurgery unit and the surgeons were on standby, waiting to operate on John's brain tumour. He also explained how dangerous it was to transport a patient in John's condition.

My pulse was racing. I looked at John and imagined he had a ticking time bomb in his head. That's what it felt like. We had no time to waste, but we could not afford to rush, either. My adrenalin was gushing through me, and I felt sick and dizzy and indescribably anxious.

We all travelled in separate cars to the Morriston. I can't remember who I was with; it could have been Santa Claus for all I knew at that moment in time. Nobody was allowed in the ambulance with John, and on the journey I just remember having horrible visions of him being resuscitated by paramedics, fighting for his life on his own, with nobody he loved by his side.

Paul explained to us how it was touch and go, and surviving the journey, let alone the op, would be a bonus. We were all so scared at this point. Sarah stayed pretty strong throughout, apart from the panic attack when Dr Bertelli explained about the cancer spreading. Me and my mum tried comforting her, as in her position, being pregnant, she couldn't afford to be getting in a state. It could be damaging for the baby.

John had also told Sarah earlier in the day how much he was looking forward to the new baby. It was also Lina's first birthday. None of us were even in the mind to celebrate it, bless her. All sorts of thoughts were running through our heads as we all travelled in separate cars to Morriston Hospital.

SARAH

Time stopped when I sat waiting for John to have the operation on his brain. 14 July 2009 had been the longest day of my life already, and it was nowhere near over. It was still light when we arrived at the Morriston. The sun was shining and it was a warm, balmy July evening. When John finally came back from theatre, the sun was starting to set and there was a chilly nip in the air. I can't tell you what happened as I waited. My mind was a blur; my life was on hold, just as John's was. All I know is that the waiting was painful. My brain ached and my body ached as I waited for news. It was horrific.

> We were introduced to a consultant by the name of Linda. She was excellent, very reassuring and helpful, and of the opinion that 'anything is possible'. Sarah was really concerned about when the radio could start as she knew that the tumours would grow and grow until John had radio to shrink them. Dr Bertelli had explained earlier how John's tumours had grown in 24 to 48 hours. This was alarming, because if they were growing at that rate every hour was crucial. Sarah just wanted radio or chemo – anything – done to improve the cancer, but Linda explained how it was 'one step at a time'.

SARAH

Linda stood smiling before me. 'It's gone well!' she announced. I think John had been in surgery for three or four hours, and it was about 8 p.m. My mind was scrambled with worry and I stared at Linda, taking in what she had just said and waiting for more information.

A few moments later, the surgeon who had actually performed John's operation appeared. 'I've just saved his life,' she said plainly.

I inhaled deeply. It was as if I'd stopped breathing when John had stopped breathing. I had held my breath all afternoon, and it felt like that was the first breath I had taken since.

The surgeon delivered the news in a matter-of-fact, but reassuring, manner. She went on to describe what she had done, making it sound like she was more of a plumber than a surgeon. 'We've drilled the hole and plugged the leak. The problem is fixed. I'll leave you now, I'm off to drill some more holes.'

Her words comforted me. They demystified the complicated neurosurgery John had undergone, but I wanted to find out more and I didn't want her to walk away just yet.

We were all bombarding Linda with questions. My mum asked, 'Will his brain be intact? Will he have any brain damage?' It was explained how all the functioning sensors were at the front, so he shouldn't be affected. We all just wanted to know the ins and outs of everything. Sarah asked Linda if she could see the scans, so a few of us followed her into a private room where there was a computer. She started talking us through the CAT scans. When you have a CAT scan, you go into a big tube and your body is photographed 'cut up' in slices from head to toe. Starting from the top of John's head, Linda explained that John had lots of tumours and one that was quite big at the back. This was the one that was causing so many problems, as it was close to the blood flow in and out of the brain. John's fluid was building up because around a pint of blood was coming into the head/brain, and this large tumour was so big it was blocking the flow out. When the surgeon told us she had just saved John's life, it was so surreal. Hearing those words proved to us how shockingly serious things were. We looked at the computer screen in amazement. The detail was unbelievable. From what we could see, there appeared to be around eight to ten tumours around his body. After the neurosurgeon finished explaining the scans, again we asked her a load of questions. Most were about future treatment: what happens next? She explained how there were several options, but at present John's pneumonia had to clear before they could look ahead. The drain was a temporary measure purely to keep John alive and relieve the pressure. The drain could be 'internalised', which meant put under John's skin and into his stomach, but that couldn't be considered yet, as any risk of infection could result in John contracting meningitis, which again would mean his life was hanging in the balance.

SARAH

I imagined the tumours in John's body would show up as black lumps on the scan pictures, but it was the opposite. They were like different-sized snowballs dotted around his body. I could see four or five small ones in his brain, and one big solid mass at the back, near the nape of his neck. Linda called them 'lesions' rather than tumours or lumps. The image of John's body was sliced up into sections. My eyes were immediately drawn to his head, but when I looked again I could see white dots scattered around his lungs and a big white blob in his right testicle.

When I was allowed to see John, I felt very emotional. I was grateful he was getting 'fixed', as Linda put it, and I told myself it was a good thing we had the CAT scan results, even though the X-rays looked so alarming.

John was in room number six. He was sedated, and it was a relief to see him lying calmly, not fighting pain or struggling to breathe, just sleeping. There were loads of wires attached to him and he had a tube coming out of his head, draining out fluid at the back. Machines recorded his oxygen levels and pulse, and he looked more stable than he had in days. 'He's made it,' I thought. I never allowed myself to think he would die, not really. It wasn't John's time. His time wasn't up yet, not by a long way.

We all kept everyone informed, and Big James was by now dealing with the ward managers and press officials within the hospitals and agreeing on press releases for the newspapers and TV.

Even though the news of John's cancer has only just hit all the press and TV, the world is going mad. There are fan groups and get-well messages popping up everywhere. All the clubs John has played for have a picture of him in their kit on their websites. The public support is ever-growing. All our phones are about to explode with everyone wanting to know how John is.

Wednesday, 15 July

Tuesday had been a really bad day. The fact that John's chances of survival had gone from 95 per cent on initial diagnosis to 80 per cent, and then 50–50, and then in the space of 24 hours were reduced to 'hopefully he'll make the journey to Morriston' – well, it was a mind-blowing roller coaster. Linda in ITU had explained it was going to be a roller coaster over the days, weeks and months ahead and we had to be prepared for that.

Throughout Wednesday, John was having lots and lots of visitors. Big James and Sarah were in the room with John for most of the day. Gordon Strachan and Martin O'Neill wanted to visit John when he was well enough. Every time a new person went in to see John, he would give a little groan. I can't really describe the sound, but he would kind of cry and say 'ooohhh'.

Bec and Joni came in to see John before the consultants were due to wake him. The kids were constantly asking to see John, but he would get emotional when he saw them, so it was a good idea for the kids to see John looking like he was sleeping and peaceful.

They stayed around an hour then left. Joni was getting lots of offers to go to his mates for tea and he seemed to be coping OK. Bec just wanted to be at the hospital all the time, understandably. She had competed for the school in an athletics meeting and won the second medal. We told John and he was chuffed (we could tell by his groans).

The whole family was there to support John, and many, many friends. As the day went on, his medication was reduced, he was taken off the ventilator and he opened his eyes, but he was still very groggy and disorientated. He tried to talk, but he couldn't manage much, though he did get a few words out. He asked Big James to 'promise me, don't let my kids see me like this'. James said he would keep that promise until John felt better. Everyone left in dribs and drabs, but my father stayed the night.

Thursday, 16 July

I woke up to the sound of my phone ringing, and Sarah's name appeared on my mobile. It was 7.50 a.m. I said 'hiya' and was delighted to hear it was John on the other end. As he was all wired up, it was difficult to understand what he was saying. He had the oxygen mask on and he'd pulled it to one side and it sounded like his chest was full of mucus and phlegm. John gave me a few groans, then Sarah came on the phone to explain he was asking for me. I told her I'd be straight there. I'm sure it must have been the quickest I've ever got ready – I was at the hospital by 8.10 a.m. I ran into the ITU to find Sarah and two doctors sitting in the waiting room. Sarah was crying, and they were in the middle of explaining that John had to be put back on the ventilator so he was now sedated again. Sarah and I were gutted about this. This effectively meant that everything was back on 'pause'. One of the doctors, Dave, said he had been with John and my dad all night. John was struggling with his chest and trying to take the ventilator tube out. (It's no wonder, really, because it was about the width of a pound coin in diameter and it ran right down his throat and into his chest.)

Dave went on to say how much of a fighter John was and how he was so impressed with his strength. He said, 'It's been a long time since I've seen anyone fight like that.' He explained that by 8 a.m. there wasn't really any alternative than to switch the ventilator back on, because John still couldn't manage to cough.

SARAH

Cyril was the first person I saw when I arrived at the hospital on Thursday morning. His clothes were crumpled, and he told me he had tried to sleep in the chair next to John's bed. My heart went out to him. He looked shattered.

Cyril explained that John had been restless and had barely slept throughout the night. 'I had to watch him,' Cyril said. 'I was worried sick he might pull out his ventilator pipe or rip off his wires and disconnect the machines. I couldn't leave him there, I just couldn't.'

'So you haven't slept a wink?'

'No, Sarah. To tell the truth, I tried to slip out to the waiting room at around six o'clock, once more staff started to appear on the ward. Ten minutes later, one of the doctors came to get me, saying John was calling for me.

'I ran back to his beside and John said: "DADDY – YOU STAY THERE!"'

'I looked John in the eye and told him: "YOU GO SLEEP!"'

Cyril laughed, and then we both laughed.

'That's so funny, Cyril. John must have still felt in control, even lying there. Isn't that typical?'

Moments like that stopped me going completely round the twist. Cyril's love for John was so powerful I could almost feel its strength. And, joking apart, I had faith that John's self-image, however misplaced at that point in time, would help pull him through. There was no way Big John was not coming back from this.

The consultant said they were going to phone Dr Bertelli to ask how much of a window they had to play with before they had to give radiotherapy. We were surprised to hear that there was 'no' window to play with. They had to do radio the following day, which meant transferring John under general anaesthetic, with a drain in his head and pneumonia, to Singleton, where the radio unit was. We were told this was a major operation in itself, to transfer a patient in John's condition from one hospital to another.

We had mixed emotions. On one hand we were pleased to hear that his treatment was starting back up, but then we were shocked at the urgency of having to have another lot of radio. Reality set in and we couldn't believe what was happening – it was horrific.

Throughout Thursday, we were told John would be kept under general until Friday's radiotherapy session, and then we'd take it from there. Despite this, and despite the fact that only close family were allowed at his bedside, the visitors continued to arrive.

Ben Thatcher drove all the way down from Ipswich. It took him five hours to get here. He chatted to us for about an hour or so and just wanted us all to know he was thinking of John.

Nathan Blake walked into the waiting room. He was really upset and, again, he wanted to come down to show John he was 100 per cent behind him.

I was spending about 14 hours a day at the hospital. You'd think it would be long, tiring and boring, but it wasn't, because people were telling funny stories about their experiences with John. Ben Thatcher talked about their time at Wimbledon, and Nathan Blake talked about their days playing for Wales together. John's close friends Karl, Mark, Colin, Tommy, Wayne and so many other extended friends and relatives gathered in the waiting room. The only thing missing was John and a pint: that's what all the boys were saying.

Messages were coming from all over the world. Vinnie Jones left a message on my father's mobile, and around 50,000 people joined an online fan group sending get-well-soon wishes.

SARAH

I followed the ambulance back from the Morriston to Singleton Hospital. I wanted to be with John as much as possible, just to be close to him, even though I felt so helpless and he had countless medical professionals all around him. I stood on the pavement outside the Singleton waiting for the ambulance doors to open. The journey had taken half an hour through quite heavy traffic. I couldn't wait to see John. His life had been saved, and he was moving on to another phase of his treatment. Now it was no longer a question of saving his life: treating his cancer, burning it out of his body with more radiotherapy, was the next step.

The squeak of the hinges as the doors opened on the back of the ambulance set my nerves on high alert. I was desperate to see John again, to be reassured he had not only survived the brain operation successfully, but this dangerous journey too. My eyes were on stalks and I could see nothing else but the back of the ambulance. A spaceship could have landed and aliens could have come over to say hello and I'd have been none the wiser.

I watched in silence as the paramedics prepared to lower John's stretcher to the pavement. I could see the shape of his feet now, covered with a stiff green NHS blanket. I was holding my breath, in case I accidentally breathed too hard and made a noise or did anything whatsoever to disturb this delicate manoeuvre. I knew it was delicate. I'd been told that it was highly unusual to transport a cancer patient who had just had a brain operation and a drain fitted in his skull halfway across town. The only reason they took the risk with John was because they had no choice. He needed urgent radiotherapy back at the Singleton or the tumours could grow some more and could stop his breathing all over again. It was a matter of life and death.

Now I could make out the shape of John's legs, and I saw the tips of his fingers emerge, followed by his arms, which were placed like two sticks of wood, perfectly parallel to his body, on top of the blanket.

Now John's trolley was on the pavement. His head was in a neck brace and he had tubes coming out of his mouth. There was a big black bandage around his head protecting the spot where the doctor had drilled into his skull. Even though I knew exactly what had happened to him, I gasped.

John looked like he'd been in a horrendous car accident. I wanted to rush over and hold him and kiss him. I wanted him to know that someone who loved him was right by his side, but I knew I couldn't. Everybody was moving very, very slowly around him. I took slow, tentative steps towards his trolley, to follow him inside. It was so disturbing to see him in that state, and I realised it wasn't just the fact he was sedated and surrounded by medical paraphernalia that alarmed me. John was a proud, strong man. He *is* a proud, strong man. There was something awful about how he was being wheeled inside the hospital and down the corridor, on public display. There was no other way into the radiotherapy department where he was headed, but still it seemed wrong.

People were stopping in their tracks, gaping at him open-mouthed.

'It's John Hartson.'

'Oh my God, you're right. Good luck, mate.'

Patients trailing drips and wires, shuffling unsteadily in dressing gowns and slippers, gave him the thumbs up. It was so surreal, so undignified and yet so terribly moving.

John was shorn of his strength and power, a bloodied, sick man under an NHS blanket. An image came into my mind that made tears spring from my eyes. It was that moving scene in *The Lion, the Witch and the Wardrobe*, when Aslan the lion has his mane shorn off and is facing death. His pride and strength have been cruelly removed, and he is naked on a slab, stripped of his dignity yet somehow still dignified. That was John in that moment. He was Aslan, and I felt powerless to help him fight off the bad blood and evil forces that had got him in this state. I still get flashbacks today of that scene. It will never leave me.

CHAPTER NINE

'You'll be fine when the new baby arrives'

SARAH

I felt a lot better knowing John's cancer was finally being treated. I'd been told he would have a strong double session of radiotherapy. I'd seen the machine they used; one of the nurses had kindly shown me a few days earlier. I found it helped me to know exactly what was going on, and I asked a stream of questions at every opportunity. I wanted to understand everything, even though seeing the machine was quite alarming. It was a big monster of a thing, like something out of *Star Wars*. The nurse explained how they positioned a laser so it hit certain areas at the back of John's head. I felt a pang of sorrow for John, having to go through all this, but I felt quite brave too. I visualised John as the big Celtic dragon I knew and loved, not the defeated giant I'd seen being wheeled in on the trolley. I knew he needed me to be strong, just like he was, and I was doing my very best for him. All my energy went into thinking about him getting well and willing him to make a speedy recovery. I was aware that visitors were still streaming to both hospitals, but I kept away from the waiting rooms. It probably sounds awful now, but I didn't want to use any of my energy making chitchat. I wanted to use every last drop being there for John. I was also aware that the media was following John's story closely. My mum had told me that before she and Frances set off for Scotland with Lina, she had reporters knocking on my door asking questions. She was afraid she'd said too much, but I told her not to worry. How could my mum possibly have been prepared for having to deal with the press about John in these circumstances? And with John in the state he was, I really didn't care what was being said outside the four walls of the hospital. Lina was safe with my family, and my job was to be here for John. That was all that mattered.

Friday, 17 July

After a double session of radiotherapy, John returned to the same intensive care ward at the Morriston. We were all thankful that everything went well at the Singleton. It was just like running a marathon, with a thousand hurdles on the way. After a few hours the doctors went in to review John, as they did every three to four hours or so. They said they would keep him highly sedated for the remainder of the day, as he'd been through a lot. As the day went on John began breathing for himself, but the doctors were adamant he was to be kept under sedation.

Swansea City had released a tribute shirt – a red one with 'Hartson 32' on the back. Big James went down to the Swans shop to buy a shirt for each of his three boys. They were all chuffed! All John's mates were getting their wives to run down to the club shop and by Friday afternoon they'd sold out of the letter 'H'.

John developed a lump at the back of his head. It was really big and swollen, but the doc put it down to the after-effects of the radio. Radiotherapy is so powerful it can sometimes burn the skin – it's almost like holding a light next to a piece of paper. Some people are so violently sick with it they have to stop their treatment halfway through regardless of the good it would do to them in the long run. We all knew John was so strong – if anyone could cope with the pain and the treatment, John could. It was just so hard to watch. John's improvement wasn't happening quickly enough. He'd been in hospital a full week now. The only plus we had to hold on to at this stage was that he was finally able to breathe for himself again, after three long days. He still had the tube in because doctors were too scared to take it out in case he needed it again. They explained that if they had to reinsert it there would be more risk of infection again, and John's chest appeared to be and sounded like it was clearing.

Neil Lennon phoned Daddy a couple of times and was sending all his love to John. He also said some great things about John and their time at Celtic. He told Daddy, 'You only ever make three or four friends in life, and John is one of them'. Everyone had such nice things to say about John. We all felt so proud to be part of his life.

We totally took over the waiting room – or the 'John Hartson Lounge' as we had started to call it. John's old headmaster, Tom Jones, had nipped in at one stage to see the family and check on John's progress, as had Eddie Edwards. When John's friends Colin and Emma visited, Emma started crying and Colin said, 'For God's sake don't start crying, it'll take you another two hours to put your make-up back on.' We all laughed. Silly little moments like that were keeping us all going.

Hayley had gone onto the Facebook fan page that had started up for John. 'I'm John's sister and would like to thank you all for all your support through this devastating time for John and the family . . . He is very, very ill. I'm not religious but ask every one of you to pray for John to fight this. Thank you,' she wrote.

The papers picked up this quote and there was a piece published in the *Western Mail* under the headline 'Sister's emotional appeal on site supporting John Hartson'. We were all a bit annoyed, because a family statement had been released and none of the other family members or friends were speaking to the press. Hayley wasn't to know, though, and there were no bad intentions. She was just trying to thank everyone. From then, we didn't log on to Internet sites like Facebook for fear of the press tracking anything down.

John's condition didn't change much on Friday. My dad stayed with John all through the night and Baby James also slept there, and I popped back up between 11.30 p.m. and 1.30 a.m., then left everyone to sleep. John had a peaceful night.

SARAH

Bags and bags of mail had started arriving for John every day. When I was on my own at home at night, I started reading through them. Even though I was physically exhausted, I was finding it impossible to switch my mind off. I thought reading the post and choosing some cards and messages to show to John would give me something constructive to do and would give him a real boost when he came round. People had really taken time to write long letters and poignant messages. They talked about their own experiences of cancer, and I was moved to tears by many of them. Some urged John to read Lance Armstrong's autobiography when he was better, to see how you can really beat testicular cancer and go on to achieve great things. Others said the experience would be ultimately life-enhancing. It would make John appreciate life more. I was constantly running different scenarios through my head, like a series of computer programs taking my mind down different paths. Ultimately, they all led to the same ending. I imagined John being better, and I was thinking thoughts like: 'We'll live life one day at a time. We'll make the most of every second. I'll never nag him again, I promise!' Reading the cards made me reflect. I didn't want to dwell on the past, but I couldn't help thinking back over John's health in the last few years. I thought about his snoring problem and his weight and picked over the 'what ifs', nearly driving myself mad. What if he'd had treatment when he first found that lump? Had that been part of his trouble at West Brom, the cause of his sleeping and tiredness and fitness issues? Could I have done more to prevent this outcome? All these thoughts ran though my mind, but I quickly told myself it didn't matter; I couldn't afford to waste energy on them. All that mattered now was the here and now. I chose the most uplifting cards and messages I could and put them in an envelope. I also packed a piece of music to play to John – the Kings of Leon's 'Use Somebody'. It was something we both liked and often listened to in the car. John's a great singer, and I pictured him singing along, like he usually did. The focus had to be on helping John wake up and helping him stay positive, getting him back on his feet and running around again like he normally did – just like the lyrics of the song. Nothing else mattered.

Saturday, 18 July 2009

They reduced John's sedation all Saturday morning, and by around 11 a.m. John was off sedation all together. John started responding at about 2.30 p.m. My dad and Sarah were with him. He was squeezing their hands and opening his eyes a bit, but he couldn't see. We were all asking questions such as, 'Can you squeeze our hands if you're in pain?' We were probably doing his head in, as no doubt everyone who went in asked the same thing over and over! It was so nice to see him responding, as we were all missing him so much.

Again, the waiting room was packed out. Brian Hamel (John's mate, a football agent), had met with John Terry and he'd sent John a message on a number-six England shirt. The support was really overwhelming.

Andy Legg also visited. He wanted to give John some inspiration, as he himself had beaten throat cancer some years previously.

Tony Thorpe had also been down for a couple of days – I think he topped and tailed with Karl!

Hundreds of cards were being sent to the hospital and all of our houses, and we were keeping them for John.

The ward manager at one point called Sarah and myself to one side, saying the florist had loads of flowers on order for John and was asking what should they do with them. We said to stagger them over the next few days; we'd sort them out from there. Just to see the tributes and get-well wishes John was receiving proved to us how much he'd touched so many people's lives and how everyone loved him.

Bec was at the hospital most days, and it was awful seeing her so worried, but just being there she felt closer and a big part of it all. She understood that she couldn't go in until her dad was a little bit better. Joni was happier playing in his mates' houses, having tea with them.

I found out that on the day John stopped breathing little Joni was praying in the garden, love him. Bless, what on earth must have been going through his little mind? Bec was asking questions and looking for reassurance, but Joni was quite silent. When we told Mam about what Joni had done, Mam said that's exactly what John would have done when he was that age, if he had seen Cyril in hospital, say. I thought of little Bec, Joni and Lina's faces and knew that John had so much to live for, especially now with the news of Sarah being due to have another baby.

SARAH

I had mixed feelings seeing John come off sedation. It took a few hours for the drugs to wear off and for him to start coming round. I desperately wanted to talk to him and ask him how he felt and tell him he was going to get better, but I had no idea how he would respond. I held his hand constantly, asking him to squeeze mine if he could hear me. I could detect the tiniest movement in one finger to begin with. I remember thinking that Lina's wee fingers had more power in them than John's. He had lost a lot of weight, too. His skin was sort of deflated on his body and his eyes were sunken. If I had to guess I'd say he'd lost about two stone, but I comforted myself with the fact that still left him around seventeen stone, so he hadn't exactly faded away. I tried to put a positive spin on everything. It wasn't a conscious decision; it was just the way I reacted. Being pregnant played a big part in my reaction, I think. I instinctively knew I couldn't break down and just fall over, because it wouldn't be good for the baby, and John needed this baby to help pull him through.

'I can feel your fingers moving, John,' I said cheerfully. 'I know you can hear me.' I played the Kings of Leon and detected a slight movement in his right eyebrow. 'Do you like it, John? Do you remember when we sang this together that night in Stratford?' Two fingers pressed very feebly into my palm. 'Remember my birthday party at Mortons in Dickens Heath? Wasn't that a great night?' His eyebrow moved again, and I carried on plucking good memories out of my head.

'Remember your 31st birthday in Glasgow, when you scored the winner against Hearts?' John's eyebrows both edged a little higher up his forehead, so I tried to remember every last detail of that day for him. 'It was 5 April 2006. You told me if you scored a goal against

Hearts at Parklands it would guarantee Celtic a place in the Premiership, even though it was early on in the season. You were opening birthday cards before the match and sorting out tickets for your mates, moaning as usual that there were never enough go round! I was planning a celebration meal for us all afterwards. When the match kicked off I was as nervous as a kitten, I don't mind admitting. But it only took you four minutes, John. Just four minutes into the game you scored the winner, and the crowd went wild. I think you smashed the ball past the Hearts goalie, Craig Gordon. Am I right? You know how clueless I am about football, but I was so proud of you. I *am* so proud of you.'

John's eyes flickered open very slowly. 'Can you see me, John?' There was no response, not even a squeeze of the hand. His eyelids were open, but his eyes were just staring out of his face.

'The celebrations started on the pitch, and we carried them out into the city and partied all night long. I felt so proud being on your arm. It felt like everyone in Glasgow was singing your name and shaking your hand. There was a power cut in the restaurant, do you remember? We ended up outside on the street. Literally thousands of people chanted your name, John. "There's only one Johnny Hartson." So many people love you. You're a hero and a fighter. We all love you.'

I'd like to say we had one of those moments like you do in films when the patient opens his eyes and suddenly your world lights up and you kiss him and he tells you he loves you. But it was nothing like that. Victoria and Cyril and Big James were also taking turns to talk to John and get him to respond, but it was clearly going to be a long process. He was slipping back in and out of sleep, and his responses were very slow. He was still extremely ill indeed.

I looked around the hospital room and felt acutely sorry for John. This was going to be his home for a good wee while yet, but he had no idea where he was. It was a private room, and he had a TV and a window looking out on some trees. I'd propped up some cards and displayed messages from football clubs and other players on John's bedside locker, as I knew when he saw them they would give him a terrific boost and remind him how highly he was thought of. I willed him to wake up, smile and enjoy reading the cards, but that moment felt a long way off. John could have been in America for all he knew. He had been transported here under sedation, and it would be a long time before he was back to his old self. I didn't want to leave his side. I thought about how frightening it would be to be in John's position, waking up in a strange room, attached to tubes and drips and with a huge ventilator pipe down your throat. It was a horrible reminder of how John had stopped breathing, and the fact it was still there made me uneasy. How would John himself feel when he became more aware of it? Even though John was now breathing unaided, the doctors would not remove the pipe yet for fear he might need it again. He was not out of the woods by any stretch. We all needed to be patient.

John remained off sedation all Saturday and Saturday evening and continued to squeeze hands for signalling, along with opening his eyes, but through signalling he said he couldn't see us.

Big James stayed the night, and by the time I arrived back in the hospital around 12.30 a.m. Big James was sleeping in the chair with a pen in his mouth. I didn't bother disturbing him; I just went in to John and sat with him until about 2.45 a.m. He was back on sedation, which I wasn't particularly happy with. Was he just being kept quiet through the night? I kept asking one particular nurse loads of questions. I think I was doing her head in, but to be honest I couldn't care less, because while John couldn't talk we had to be his voice. Even though I know doctors and nurses try their best, to them it's a job and John's a number. But to us he meant the world and we *needed* him – every single one of us.

Any time any of us went in to John, we kept telling him that he had to keep fighting. We were really hoping that he wanted to keep fighting. All the doctors told us that they hadn't seen such a determined person for a long time, which proved to all of us he wanted to fight.

Mark and Paul had gone in to see him on Saturday night, and he held both their hands, pulled them close to his chest and gave them both a thumbs up.

John gave me a little squeeze before I left the hospital at 2.45 a.m., and to be honest I cried all the way home, because I just didn't have a good feeling about leaving, but I had been falling asleep by John's bed side and I started jumping as I was falling asleep and waking John!

I was OK when I got home, because he was in the best hands and I needed to accept he would eventually get better. I wanted him to run before he could crawl. It was a long process.

SARAH

I pulled over at the all-night garage for petrol on my way home from the hospital. The early editions of the Sunday newspapers had already arrived. The only time I had ever bought papers at that time in the morning was when John had scored a winner and hit the headlines, and we'd picked up a copy after a night of celebrating so he could read the back pages and have a good souvenir to remember his triumph. Now I picked up a copy of the *News of the World* with a heavy heart. I knew the press had been following John's progress all week and they were bound to carry a story. I flicked though it before I restarted the engine, and my eyes fell on a thick black headline: 'Secret Baby Joy For Tragic Soccer Ace John Hartson – Cancer Victim May Not Live to See Birth'. I reread it again and then my eyes dropped to the first paragraph of the story: 'Cancer-ravaged soccer hero John Hartson's girlfriend is pregnant with a baby he may never live to see . . .' Tears sprang from my eyes, but I wiped them away angrily. 'What a load of rubbish,' I said, throwing the paper on the back seat. 'What an absolute load of nonsense.' It hurt, though. It stung me inside, and I smoothed my hands over my stomach and told our baby that everything would be OK, because Daddy was a fighter, and Daddy *was* going to live to see his baby.

Sunday, 19 July

John was on 10 ml of sedation through the night, and it was then put up to 15 ml. We were disappointed every time John's sedation was increased, because we so desperately wanted him to wake and come off the tubes. Any time any of us saw John we kept saying, 'Just hang on in there – you'll be off the tube soon.' We didn't have a clue, really, nor could we possibly imagine what thoughts were running through his head. He was probably thinking, 'Shut up – what do you know!' But we all kept saying, 'Keep fighting.' We were all trying to be positive.

We were told John was going to have another load of radio tomorrow, and we suspected they would keep John on sedation throughout the day, as he was due to go to Singleton again in the morning.

Work had been great with us. I was on compassionate leave, and Daddy said he never wanted to work again! I'm sure that was heat of the moment, but he just wanted to spend the next months helping John out, then enjoying being with John once he'd made a full recovery.

At around 11.15 a.m., Mam, Dad and Big James went down to the hospital chapel, where there was a traditional Sunday service. The chaplin mentioned John and they also sang 'Calon Lân'. My mother said it was giving her strength. She also told me that on the Tuesday night, which was John's worst day, our family vicar Gareth Hopkin had visited John's bedside and said a beautiful prayer.

Everyone I spoke to was saying prayers for John and texting me to say they had mentioned John in their church today. It was so nice to know so many people were thinking of him.

John didn't really respond right through the day and evening as they increased his sedation, and by the night he was on 25 ml. Daddy slept the night.

Monday, 20 July

Everyone was telling us how Lance Armstrong had had exactly the same as John – their conditions were identical – so we hung on to the hope that someone else had beaten it, so surely John could beat it. Lance Armstrong had been leaving messages for John on Twitter. Thousands more were joining support groups on the likes of Facebook. It was overwhelming. We couldn't wait until John was conscious and aware of the support; it would be such a boost of encouragement.

SARAH

On Monday morning I woke up early and realised I'd slept soundly, and I felt surprisingly recharged. Perhaps it was adrenalin mixing with my pregnancy hormones. I had a sense that we had entered a new phase in John's recovery and it was time to really push forward and fight. Today he was having more radiotherapy, but I knew the routine now and it didn't scare me. I welcomed it, because I knew it was making John better. It was amazing how quickly the hospital routine had become second nature. My life had been turned upside down, but I felt it was also in some kind of order now that John's treatment was progressing. I had a mental checklist in my head: Today, radiotherapy; tomorrow, maybe we could get rid of that ventilator pipe down his throat.

The radiotherapy would deal with the brain tumours; then surely it would be a simple question of starting up the chemotherapy. Then we'd really be in business. John would be as right as rain before we knew it. Chemo would kill off any other random cancer cells and mop up the tumours on his lungs. He'd have to have his testicle removed at some point, of course, but that seemed a minor formality now.

I spoke to my mum and Frances on the phone. Lina was having a fine old time up in Scotland. I missed her like mad, but I was relieved she was away, being taken care of. I didn't like being on my own in the house, especially at night, but at the same time I couldn't have coped with visitors or anything else at all in my life. I was functioning quite well in the circumstances, just trying to eat properly and get enough sleep. Being as useful as possible when I was sitting with John and watching over him, and looking after our unborn child: they were the priorities.

From knowing next to nothing about cancer, I was learning fast. I quizzed the doctors at every opportunity. When John was taken back to Singleton again on Monday morning, I asked more questions. One doctor told Victoria and I that radio is so powerful it can leave burn marks on the skin, and some people get so ill with it they have to stop the treatment halfway through. I knew John would cope. Don't ask me how I knew, but I did. There was no way he wouldn't be strong enough

169

to take it. His strength was one of his distinguishing characteristics. I thought about how he had lifted up me and Lina a few weeks earlier in the kitchen. I had her in my arms, and he hugged me and lifted us both up, as if we were a couple of plastic dolls. I thought about how he always teased me about overstuffing my holiday suitcases. It was true. Once, they felt laden with bricks and I couldn't budge them an inch, but John picked them up without turning a hair. I felt safe when he was around. I felt protected from the world, and I felt we could do anything together, because he was my big strong powerhouse of a man.

By this stage it had been decided that only myself, Cyril and Diana should visit John's bedside. After showing some initial flickers of response, John was heavily sedated again and was not responding. We were all worried about the risk of him catching more infections and taking another step backwards, so it didn't make sense for him to have more visitors than necessary, especially when he wouldn't even know they were in the room. Cyril and Diana came in and out regularly, but I sat for hours, just looking at John and chatting to him. Cyril usually stayed the night at the hospital, which was a great comfort to me and I'm sure to John, too.

When John was settled back after his latest radiotherapy and we were all alone, I talked to him about our new baby.

'I've spoken to the midwife and she is booking me in for our first scan,' I told him. 'Do you remember how exciting it was when we were expecting Lina? Won't it be brilliant to see the scan pictures?

'Also I have some great news, John. Because of what happened at Lina's birth, they will probably book me in for a routine Caesarean. We won't have to go through another delivery nightmare or any emergencies – it'll be a breeze by comparison.

'Do you think it will be another wee girl? I'd love it if it was; I really would. I can't imagine having a boy. Besides, we've got a house full of pink plastic! I'm sure it's a wee girl. Lina will love being a big sister. She is fine, by the way, having a ball running my family ragged in Scotland.

'We'll all be home together soon – you, me and Lina. You'll be fine when the new baby arrives.'

I probably sounded a bit silly, chatting away as animatedly as I could and just hearing my own voice bouncing back off the walls, but I didn't care. I was sure the best way to get John to respond and fight was to be positive and remind him what a great life he had waiting for him.

I tried to pluck footballing memories out of my mind, too. I reminded him about the framed Golden Boot from Celtic on the wall of our office at home, and the red Wales shirt John once wore, emblazoned with messages from other players.

'You're a real hero, John,' I told him. 'All the Wales fans are rooting for you, and all the Celtic fans too, of course. Tens of thousands of people are leaving messages of support on the Internet. All the clubs you've played for have tribute pages posted up.

'I will try to name them all – now there's a challenge for me. OK, let me get this right – you've played for so many clubs I've lost track. Let me see: Luton, Arsenal, West Ham, Wimbledon, Coventry, Celtic, West Brom. Am I right, John? You know I'm not the most knowledgeable person when it comes to football!'

John breathed steadily, and I could detect his eyeballs moving beneath the sallow skin of his eyelids.

'I remember when you told me about playing for Wales, John, and I hung on your every word. You described your most memorable game. It was against Finland and you were 27 years old – so I'm guessing it must have been 2002. Gosh, that's seven years ago, John, but I know you remember it like it was yesterday.

'Mark Hughes was your manager, and you were playing in the European Championship qualifiers. See, I do listen when you talk about football! You scored, John. Wales won 2–0 and you scored, setting your country off to a flying start. Then you beat Italy at the Millennium Stadium in Cardiff. Do you remember the Welsh crowd singing their hearts out in full voice? You told me it made your heart sing. People all over Wales, all over the world, in fact, are rooting for you now, John.'

Tuesday, 21 July

Around elevenish, John went down for his last session of radio. We began to learn how things worked, and as far as we knew it all went well. I returned to work even though my mind wasn't on it, but in fairness I'd had ten days off, and work told me I could be flexible with my hours. There was no chance of Daddy going back to work – he was spending all of his time at the hospital. Friends helped take care of his business. All our friends were offering help; the offers were flooding in from everywhere. Anna, across the road from Mam's house, was doing Mam's ironing and a bit of cooking for them. Everyone wanted to do their bit and show support.

Karl would arrive at the hospital every day with different things: sandwiches, cherries, sweets. Every day he would arrive with a different kind of food. We wondered what made him decide what to bring each day!

Old friends of my parents and people who had been close to John throughout his childhood visited the waiting room. John would have loved to have seen so many old faces and have a chat. It was such a shame he wasn't well enough at this stage to see people, but we hoped soon enough he would be. Some friends, like Paul Glover, spent a lot of time at the hospital but didn't really want to see John. They would get upset and didn't want to see him until he was sitting up and eating grapes. John remained on sedation through the night. I know we were being a bit naïve, but we thought, 'If John's had all his radiotherapy, why can't they wake him up straight away?' The doctors kept telling us it was like a marathon or a roller coaster, but we all found it difficult to handle. We were impatient. We just wanted John out of hospital, and well.

Wednesday, 22 July

John was quite uncomfortable. He was pulling on his ventilator tube and heaving and gagging, and seemed to be in quite a bit of pain. Nothing anyone did was helping, really. We were getting worried, as we had hoped John would start to feel better. He was only opening his eyes a little and just didn't seem like he wanted to wake up. Mam and I didn't think John had much fight in him. There was talk of John having a tracheotomy so he could get rid of the tube in his mouth, but nothing was happening quickly enough. A lot of the time we wanted to shout from the rooftops, 'What the hell is happening?' He was like a zombie and we were his voice, but we also had to remain calm and respectful. We were all impatient and looking for a miracle, but nothing was happening.

Some days I woke up and wondered whether this was a dream. Then after a few minutes I'd realise it was far from a dream – my brother was critically ill. There were times when I think all the family were in a state of shock . . . but just trying to put on a brave face.

Thursday, 23 July

My father phoned me first thing and said John hadn't had a particularly good night. He'd been hallucinating a lot and was finding it difficult to breathe. We hoped the tracheotomy would be carried out today as we thought that while John was having so much discomfort with this big thick tube down his throat he wouldn't really want to wake up. When he was even partially awake with the tube in his mouth, he would be gagging on it. It made him heave – the feeling must be the worst in the world! My dad was really concerned on the phone. He also said that when he got changed last night he'd left all his money in his other trousers, so he hadn't had a cup of tea all through the night. I took some money up to him and we went for a cup of tea. We didn't really know why John was so confused and hallucinating again – he was hardly talking or opening his eyes. It was like a vicious circle. When John woke up and was confused, they'd sedate him again. It was so frustrating, as all we wanted was for John to wake up, come round and not be confused. We had to rely on the expertise of the nurses, and if we were frustrated, God knows how poor John felt.

John went down for the tracheotomy around 3 p.m. and it all went well. We were all nervous about it, and it sounded really awful to have your throat cut, but if it meant not having that awful tube in your mouth surely it would make a difference?

He started to come round a few hours after the tracheotomy. A few of us went in to see him: Dad, Sarah and Mam. It was about 7.30 p.m. John's eyes were open a little and he was kind of lip-talking. No sound would come from John's mouth, as there was effectively air in the passage with the hole from the tracheotomy, but we could lip-read a little. He was confused and asking Sarah who she was sleeping with and pointing at some of the male nurses and saying, 'Him!' The next minute he was saying they were finished; then a minute later he was talking about other things.

I was worried about why John was so confused. I thought he might be having a reaction to one or more of the medicines he was on. I even considered talking to the doctors about changing his medication, until Big James told me to leave it to the experts. (Ha ha – I'd learned so much about cancer in the last two weeks I really did think I was an expert – ha ha!)

SARAH

When John started hallucinating again, it was very distressing. In my mind that stage was over, and we should have been moving on to the next phase of his treatment, not going backwards. When he was still and quiet, it was no relief. His eyes were rolling; they looked like they weren't part of him. There was no life in his eyes, no life in him. It was terrifying to see him like that.

I looked around at all the tubes and wires, the beeping machines and the huge dressing on the back of John's head. He was clearly still in a very bad way, but I still never allowed myself to think he wouldn't get better. I couldn't let myself go down that road. It wasn't John's time – his time wasn't anywhere near up yet.

'I know you're sleeping with him,' he suddenly said. He was red in the face and coughing with the effort of spitting the words out. Because of the tracheotomy he sounded like some sort of alien. It was very alarming, but I had gone beyond the stage of being embarrassed like I was when he first said these things soon after he was admitted. It's amazing how cancer impacts on you. It gives you a whole new perspective on the world, and inconsequential things like my embarrassment didn't matter at all.

'It's not true, John,' I said gently. It was difficult to know what to say.

174

I didn't want to upset him by telling him he was off his head on drugs, but I wanted to put his mind at rest. Whenever one particular male nurse appeared, John gave him a hell of a time. 'Don't worry, I've seen it all before,' he said politely. John is normally such a gentleman. I felt so sorry for him being so out of control.

It had been a frustrating few days, with virtually no progress being made in John's recovery, and I left the hospital with a heavy heart on Thursday night. It was disturbing seeing John so distressed and confused, and I knew the best thing all round was to say goodbye for the night and tell John I would see him in the morning. Hopefully that way he would get a better night's sleep, and perhaps if I wasn't there, there may be less chance of him hallucinating and getting himself worked up.

It was only about 11 p.m. when I got home, went into the office and switched on the computer. I thought I might have a look at some websites that could give me some information about testicular cancer, or perhaps take a look at some of the club websites that were supporting John. Really, I just wanted something to feed my busy mind. It was racing, and I wanted to channel my energy somehow, but I didn't really know where to start.

I pressed a couple of buttons, and suddenly the screen looked like the windscreen of my car when it was hammering it down with rain. The tears just flooded out of my eyes, and I dropped my head in my hands and sobbed. I heard a tap on the window and it made me jump. When I turned to look it was Brenda, my neighbour who lives opposite. 'I saw you crying through the window, Sarah. Shall I come and sit with you?'

I let her steer me to the kitchen, and we drank hot tea. It was a comfort to be able to chat freely for a little while, away from the hospital and in the safety of my own kitchen. At times, the hospital felt very claustrophobic. I realised I watched what I said, because I tried to protect other people from getting too upset, and I also wanted to protect John's privacy. Sometimes I felt uncomfortable when some of his intimate personal information – scan results, reports about his mental state and so on – were discussed freely in the corridors by well-meaning friends and visitors. We'd heard stories about reporters dressing up as porters to sneak into the hospital to see him, too. Whether it was true or not, I don't know, but it added to the stifling atmosphere in the hospital.

'Thanks,' I said to Brenda, 'I feel a lot better, I'll get some sleep now.' When she walked back over the road, waving at me and smiling, I remembered what it felt like to be, well, just normal again for a little while. I wanted my old life back, with John back in my arms.

When I lay in bed, I filled my head with the small piece of good news I had heard that day. The doctors said it shouldn't be long before they could operate to 'internalise' the drain in John's head. At the moment he still had that tube coming out leading to a bottle. It wasn't pleasant to look at, as it was basically John's brain fluid and it was a horrible yellowy kind of liquid. The operation to internalise it would not be carried out until John's pneumonia had cleared up completely, so it seemed the doctors felt his infection had nearly gone. Internalising the drain would be another big operation – the fluid would be fed down into his stomach instead of into the bottle. It sounds quite horrific when I explain it now, but at the time I welcomed it. It proved John was actually getting better, and it would take him one step closer to being able to have chemotherapy.

Chapter Ten

'This will be my last night'

Friday, 24 July

John was in and out of sleep, and Sarah and my dad were in and out of John's room, but Sarah spent most of the day in with him. I went in about teatime with Mam, and it was lovely to see John awake, yet worrying that he was still so confused. The doctors had told my dad and Sarah that when they had time later, they would go through the results of the chest X-rays. They also said John's chest looked clearer and the phlegm was now moving up from his chest to his throat, which was a good sign, as it meant the infection was clearing and chemo would be able to start. Physiotherapists were going in to see John daily and were working on the crap in his chest.

There was a picture in the paper of the Cardiff v. Celtic game at Cardiff's new stadium. Celtic had brought a flag down with 'Big John – You're Always in Our Hearts' written on it. It was about 50 feet long and the picture showed it travelling around the stadium. My cousin Mark said all the Cardiff supporters were even singing 'there's only one Johnny Hartson' all through the game. We all wondered what John would think about Cardiff City fans chanting his name. It was certainly a change from the usual chants John had from Cardiff fans!

I saw John for a short while, and he was pretty quiet. When I was leaving, I told John I'd send Big James in. I gave John a kiss and told him I'd see him tomorrow, and then I told Big James to go in.

When Big James went in to see John, he was really low. He told James he couldn't fight any more. He said he'd had enough. 'This will be my last night,' he said. 'I'm losing the battle.' James struggled to convince him otherwise. James came out of the room and went to talk to Sarah.

SARAH

I was shocked when James relayed John's words to me. My John is a fighter, not a quitter. I knew it was just an emotional reaction, or perhaps it was even the drugs talking. I didn't for a second believe John really felt like giving up. He had so much to live for. Earlier that day he had managed to whisper to me a little. 'When I am better we'll get married,' he said. 'I'll be out of here to help you when you have the baby. I want to live to see my baby.' I focused on positive, fun things, like places we would visit, holidays we would have and how pretty Lina would be as our little flower girl, with her blonde curls. I tried not to let him get too emotional, because when he got worked up he coughed and spluttered, and blood as well as the yellow brain fluid squirted out of the drain in his head. I felt very strongly that he needed to be wrapped in cotton wool emotionally. I said 'yes' to everything he said. If he'd asked me to fly to the moon with him when he got out of hospital, I'd have agreed.

For whatever reason, when James went in, John gave vent to those dark thoughts I had tried to suppress. James relayed his conversation with tears in his eyes. He was distraught; we all were.

John must have been feeling so weak. When I went in later, I noticed he could hardly move his arms and legs and was so slow – it was as if his whole body was on shutdown.

Everything was so up and down. You'd leave the hospital and everyone was on a high, then you'd phone a couple of hours later and everyone seemed so depressed again. All of our lives had come to a halt, and it was hard to shut off when you left the hospital – you'd take it with you everywhere.

SARAH

That night, the doctors gave John temazepam to help him rest and go to sleep. It seemed to work, and John calmed down a lot and drifted off to sleep. Again, Cyril stayed the night, and I went home with a heavy heart. Sleeping alone, I thought about our wedding plans. We'd talked about having a summer wedding, perhaps in July 2010. I told myself that might fit in perfectly with me having the baby in March. I'd have chance to shape up and plan after the birth. It would be perfect, in fact. I desperately wanted to be married to John, and I didn't let his condition throw me off track. It was something I'd wanted for years, and now I wanted it more than ever. Cyril was John's official next of kin, and he was the person who signed the consent forms for John's operations. That pained me. I was pregnant with John's child and we were engaged to be married, but I was not officially tied to John, and it didn't feel right. I wanted to wear his ring on my finger and promise to take care of him, in sickness and in health. I wanted to press a fast-forward button and walk down the aisle with John and tell him that I would love him come hell or high water. I pictured him wearing a kilt at our wedding. I'd teased him that he'd have to wear a kilt, as he was marrying a Scot, and John being John, he had actually agreed. 'As long as I can pick a Welsh tartan,' he said. 'And am I allowed to go commando style?' he joked. When I drifted off to sleep, I clung on to those hopes and dreams. 'There's no way he won't make it,' I told myself.

Saturday, 25 July

The doctors confirmed that John would be having his operation to internalise the drain at some point this afternoon, and Dr Martin, a highly qualified neurosurgeon, would be carrying out the op.

Again my dad signed the consent form, and it was a bit of a wake-up call each time John had to have an op. All the risks were highlighted in these forms, and it really was a bit of a reality check. We were told the op would last between an hour and an hour and a half, but it would take as long as it takes, so to speak.

My dad seemed pretty down. He looked tired, and everything was getting on his nerves. He was worried sick about John. He told us on so many occasions how much he'd rather he were the one in the bed.

Dave (one of the doctors) was really good at explaining things. He'd give examples of the war days — he would say things like, 'We've all got cancer cells in our body, but as they grow, the soldiers on the front line shoot them dead. However, what's happened with John is that one bad cell' — or, as Dave called it, 'the enemy' — 'has hidden away and the soldiers couldn't find it, and it's planted itself and set up home in one place and grown and grown. In John's case this was in his testicle.' John needed chemo to help beat off the cancer that had spread to other areas of his body, but he wasn't fit enough at present. What the chemo would do is insert poisonous chemicals into John's body, but these chemicals would also kill the good soldiers, and John needed all the good soldiers at the moment to kill off infection and so on.

John would take a liking or disliking to some doctors and nurses. Dave spent a lot of time in there, along with Dawn, who John seemed to like, but there were some staff John didn't like, and he wasn't shy in telling them, either. The doctors said a bit of paranoia was common, and my dad also explained that John was not normally rude and he was the nicest, kindest person ever, and when he came out of this he would revisit the ward and give them all a big hug.

A big blue envelope arrived for John. It seemed like there was a card inside, so my dad told me to open it. We opened the wrapper to reveal this big picture of John in his Arsenal kit, with the words 'Thinking of You' on top. When we opened the card, there were loads of messages from everyone sending their best regards and get-well messages to John. It seemed as if a lot of the messages were from people who had known John when he was playing for Arsenal. We thought it was so nice of everyone to make such an effort. On the right-hand side it said: 'Keep fighting, John. The boys are in pre-season, but we're all wishing you well. Arsène and the boys.' The manager of Arsenal and a living legend was sending John his love – if only John knew, it would be such a boost! It was so nice of them to do that.

SARAH

I pushed a trolley round Tesco's. I brushed my teeth and I paid the gas bill. I emptied the bins and waved at neighbours when I drove down the road. All the mundane things in life that just don't stop, no matter what, probably kept me sane. I checked our bank account, too. In fact, that was something that wasn't as mundane as you might think. Of course, John's freelance TV pundit work had come to an abrupt halt, and I needed to make sure we didn't have any immediate cash-flow problems. I wasn't unduly worried. The *Scottish Sun* had very generously agreed to keep paying John for his weekly football column for the time being. It was not only a weight off my mind knowing there was still cash coming in, but it was also a great show of support for John, and it demonstrated how highly they thought of him. When I checked over our accounts I thought I had a pretty good idea what to expect, but in fact I got a nasty shock. There were debits for £1,000 here and £1,000 there that I couldn't account for. The further back I looked, the more black holes I found. I was in no fit state mentally to start picking over our accounts in detail, so I called our financial advisor and expressed my concerns. When I finished the call, I sat motionless. I knew I didn't need an expert to tell me what was going on. Despite John's promises and good intentions, he had continued to gamble. No doubt he told himself he could get away with the odd little flutter because we could afford it and nobody would get hurt. I'd heard that line a thousand times. His TV work was flooding in. He was earning different amounts each month, so it must have been easy to 'lose' a chunk of cash here and there. What with the pregnancy and Lina still being so small, I hadn't made time to check the accounts as thoroughly as I should have. I felt sick – not because of the money, but because of John's disappointing behaviour. He had gone against his agreement to stick to his set spending allowance and must have used a cash card I knew nothing about. I looked around our home, at our four walls, and I felt a little scared. We had no idea how long it would take John to recover. That was the priority, not the money. But at the same time, we couldn't sweep this under the carpet. John needed his home more than ever. Coping with financial problems and worrying about paying the mortgage on top of everything else was just unthinkable. It frightened me, and I tried to suppress panic as I wondered how we would cope. Perhaps I could go back to work as a teacher to help support us while John convalesced? Just the thought of it made me feel like another weight had been strapped on my back, and I felt like crying. I felt a flash of anger, too. John should have been a multi-millionaire, with all the money he had earned. It never bothered me before, because we never had to worry about money. I didn't demand a lavish lifestyle, I just wanted us all to be comfortable, but now I felt vulnerable and afraid.

I clenched my fists and bit my lip.

'Stop,' I told myself firmly. 'Get real, Sarah. There are plenty of people worse off. You've spotted the leak now. It isn't going to drown you.'

I tried to convince myself that maybe this would prove to be one good thing to come out of John's illness. Maybe, at long last, John would give up his gambling habit. My mind flicked back to him lying in hospital. I couldn't possibly be angry with him, not now. He had an addiction, a weakness. But it was his only weakness. He was tough and strong, and today was the day he was going to get stronger still.

I walked into Lina's room and realised I hadn't been in there for over a week. The soft white duvet on her cot was still ruffled from the last time she'd slept there, and the familiar smell of talcum powder and baby wipes made my heart skip a beat. I missed Lina so much. I wanted her back home with her daddy. I wanted all three of us back home together. A nurse had asked me if Lina owned one of those Etch A Sketch toys, where you can write on the screen and then shake the pad to clear it and start again. John's tracheotomy had been successful, but his voice was very weak and he couldn't talk properly, so it was suggested he might be able to jot things down instead. I found an Etch A Sketch pad still in its package. Lina was too little to use it just yet, but at least it might help John communicate while he got used to having the pipe in his throat.

Everything had gone well with the op to internalise the drain, and we were all over the moon. John's tracheotomy had been a success, too. His voice box would now be affected; therefore over the next few days he might need to write messages with the Etch A Sketch. They tried it out, but it wasn't very dignified, if I'm honest. John didn't really have the strength and coordination to use it, so instead they made arrangements to have a microphone fitted on the end of his tracheotomy pipe. Whenever anyone has a tracheotomy they lose the full use of their voice box, as it effectively has a hole in it and the vocal chords are not able to vibrate as usual. The microphone helped a bit, and it was nice to hear some sort of sound coming out of John, even though he sounded quiet and a bit funny, and still a bit confused. He was convinced I worked there at the Morriston hospital.

Sunday, 26 July 2009

Daddy phoned around 10 a.m. to say John had had his best night's sleep yet. He did have some temazepam to help him get off to sleep around 5 a.m., but he was resting lovely. My dad had slept there again and had been in and out with John. At one point in the middle of the night John was sleeping, but Dawn had to wake him up to do the regular checks. She said to my dad, 'My heart is telling me to leave him to sleep, but the neurosurgeons have told me to wake him up.'

John said to Daddy around 5.30 a.m., 'I can feel me getting stronger, Dad. I feel like going for a walk with you.'

Dawn said, 'I don't think you are quite ready for that yet, John.'

Then John said, 'Well, maybe just down the corridor and back then.' He still had a great sense of humour, which was surprising after what he was going through.

SARAH

The moment I arrived on the ward, I could sense a shift in the air. Cyril had gone home for a bath and a couple of hours' sleep, and I knew that meant John must be in a better state, because Cyril would not have left the hospital otherwise. I pushed the door open into John's room and was thrilled to see him propped up against his pillows in bed. He looked worn out but managed a small, slow smile. A nurse came in and told me they were going to move him into the chair by his bed and try to give him some ice cream at about 11 a.m., which would be the first thing he'd eaten for himself in weeks. 'Can I have it now?' John asked. He sounded like a little boy, and I didn't know whether to laugh or cry.

John's eyes were still sunken, he was unshaven and he had lost what looked like about four stone in weight by now. He was a wispy, pale shadow of the man who had staggered into the hospital weeks earlier, but he finally looked and seemed more like himself again. He had made it through the worst part, and now the only way was up.

'We'll sort it out as soon as we can,' I said to John. The nurse nodded her approval, and we asked John's cousin Mark, who was waiting outside, to fetch John some ice cream as quickly as he could.

'Where's my ice cream? Can I have it now?' John repeated.

'You're like a dog with a bone, John,' I laughed. 'Mark's gone to get some of your favourite chocolate chip. He'll be as quick as he can.'

When the ice cream finally melted on John's lips, we all smiled. He only managed the tiniest few spoonfuls, and I had to help feed him like I did with Lina, but it was a magical moment.

'I'm glad you enjoyed that,' I said, leaning over to kiss him on the cheek.

John slowly raised his hand and took hold of my arm. 'Tomorrow we'll go to La Parilla for lunch and we'll have a bottle of champagne,' he said, looking straight into my eyes. I felt like a teenager being asked out on a date. My stomach somersaulted and the blood shot up my neck and brought a glow to my cheeks.

'We'll do that when you're good and ready, John. That'll be great!'

I sat back down on the end of John's bed and let him find some more words.

'Who is here?' he asked me next. 'Is Vic still working here?'

I sighed and my shoulders tensed. I could feel John slipping very slightly away from me again. I wanted to grab him and shake him and tell him to stay, but his mind was playing tricks. 'Vic is a legal secretary, John. She's worked for the council for years. She doesn't work here in the hospital.'

'I don't believe anything you tell me,' John replied. He sounded suddenly angry now, but his expression didn't change. It was as if he was too tired to use any facial expressions. 'You tell me lies. I know you are sleeping with him. I do know, you know, Sarah. I've seen him. It's that male nurse who's always in here. I'm not stupid, you know.'

'But John, it's not true. It's just your imagination running wild. Honestly, it's not true, don't get yourself worked up, it's not going to do you any good. I love you, John. We're having another baby and getting married. I would never lie to you.'

He looked straight through me. 'I know about that doctor who comes in here. I know she is sleeping with that male nurse too. I'm gonna grass the pair of them up to her husband.'

'John, settle down and rest. I'm glad you enjoyed your ice cream. You look so much better; it's brilliant.

'Lina has been to the park with Frances and the kids, and she's had ice cream too. Like father like daughter!'

John's eyelids dropped and he fell silent.

The neurosurgeon popped his head round the door and beckoned me outside. 'I'll see you in a minute, John,' I smiled.

'I'll wait here,' John said softly.

The neurosurgeon told me that John was making better progress than they expected at this stage. I was absolutely delighted and went straight back into John's room to tell him, only to find him sleeping like a baby. There was no hint of the gruff, spluttering breathing or, indeed, any snoring at all. I sat and held his hand and just stared at him intently. I couldn't believe how much better he was, and I couldn't take my eyes off him.

I told my mam what John had said about taking Sarah to La Parilla, and I thought 'if only'. Mam said she'd *carry* him to La Parilla if only he was well enough. When we were telling my dad he'd eaten ice cream, he said, 'He'll want a chicken dinner now tomorrow.' I went in with John, but he was sleeping, so I didn't want to disturb him. I just sat holding his hand for around 15 minutes, then left him to have a nice rest. John's breathing was great. It made us all wonder whether the snoring problem John had had over the last few years was connected to the tumours.

Monday, 27 July

The media attention on John was phenomenal. Everyone was saying such nice things about him, all his old managers. He was even being offered jobs – or told to get in touch when he was well and so on. I knew this would be a big boost to John when he was told.

When I arrived at the hospital after work, I was really pleased to see Bec and Joni there. They ran to me and told me they'd seen their dad. I was chuffed. I knew this meant he was continuing to get better. For more than ten days the kids hadn't seen John, and they hadn't seen him conscious since 14 July, so it was lovely for them to be reassured and see him awake and talking. The kids had their red Swans tops on with Hartson 32 on the back, and even though we'd told John about the shirts some days before, he was shocked to see them and thought they were great.

When I went into John's room, he looked great – well, better than he had been looking. We chatted for a little while. He asked me who was in the waiting room – he liked knowing who was there. He was still convinced that I worked there in the Morriston Hospital, but other than that his confusion was getting less and less as time went on.

He told me he was so happy to see the kids and started saying how lovely they are and how beautiful Bec is – and for the first time he was actually speaking about them without getting too emotional, without crying.

SARAH

I found it incredible how we all adapted to John's changing condition. In normal circumstances, this would have been dreadful. John was still practically bed-bound. He had lost nearly five stone in weight by the time he woke up, and he didn't appear to have an ounce of strength in his body. His mind was still wandering and he was confused, and he was drifting in and out of sleep. Yet we were all delighted to see him like this. I could see my big strong John re-emerging every day, and it was fantastic. 'When will I start chemo?' he asked me. 'When can I go home?' To hear him talking about the future was completely uplifting. 'I can't wait for the baby to come.'

I always knew he had a future to look forward to, but I never dared hope it would be in his grasp as quickly as this. If John continued to remain free of infection and progress the way he had in the last day or two, the plan was to start chemo next week. He'd be moved back to Singleton and begin five consecutive days of chemo, and hopefully continue the course as an outpatient.

Wednesday, 29 July
Mid-morning, John's tracheotomy was removed. This was massive progress, as John had been on a ventilator (whether in his mouth or throat) for 15 days. Even though for some of that time John was initiating his own breathing, to be off the machine completely proved to us that the doctors were beginning to have confidence in John getting better.

Hayley and Baby James called up with a big pot of stew around 2.30 p.m. and a few tucked in – the visiting room was still never empty. John was brought out of bed and sat in the chair for 45 minutes. My dad sat and had a chat with him. John was very weak but remained positive. He was too weak to even stand on his own two feet without support, but I guess this was the physios' and doctors' way of doing things one step at a time.

My dad phoned me about midday to give me an update on John. Dad sounded down – he said he was having a bad day. He said he was going to go home, have a nice soak in the bath and a few hours to himself. I'd never heard my father like that the whole time John had been in hospital. Everyone was entitled to a bad day. My dad had been like a pillar of strength to all of us, especially John. There were people in and out of the hospital, some practically living in the hospital waiting room, and we relied on an update from my father when we weren't there, so it probably got a bit too much for him and he needed an hour or so out.

Later, I met my dad back at the hospital. He was in with John. When I walked in, John kind of raised his eyebrows as if to say 'hello'. It was just so nice to see him awake. John seemed nice and calm, more focused. Three to four days ago his movements were so slow; everything seemed to be in slow motion. Even moving his hand to his head, touching his nose – whatever he did was really slow. Today, that was so much better.

John told me he'd seen my friends (but couldn't remember their names). It was the first day he wasn't convinced I worked there at the Morriston.

My dad was talking to John about future treatment plans. John was taking it all in. He seemed to understand . . . then he said, 'I'll be home in a few days now, see, Vic.'

My dad said, 'No, John, you'll be going somewhere like Sancta Maria for convalescent care.' As much as he'd have loved to be telling John, 'Yes, you'll be home in a few days,' he knew he couldn't.

John said, 'I'll be able to live a normal life, won't I, Dad?'

My father said, 'Yes, of course you will, son. Once you get the all-clear you'll have to take care of what you eat and drink, and your exercise – but yes, there is no reason why you can't live a normal life.' My father then gave Lance Armstrong as an example. 'Look what he has gone on to achieve – and he had exactly the same as you.'

CHAPTER ELEVEN

Waking up

JOHN

How did I feel when I started to wake up and had my first lucid thoughts? Frustrated that I couldn't get out of bed. I'd lost every ounce of energy, and I felt like a totally disabled person. That's what I was. I couldn't even get myself out of bed to go to the toilet. I felt useless and worthless. The nurses were all in their 20s. They were blonde, looked fabulous and smelled gorgeous. I must have stunk something terrible, and looked even worse. So was my first clear thought, 'Will I live?' No, it wasn't. My first thought was about how embarrassed and frustrated I felt, lying there, not even being able to lift the remote control. The beautiful nurses lifted me onto a commode and emptied my bedpans, and I could have died of shame. I told them how embarrassed I was, and they said, 'It's second nature to us, don't worry about it.' I'd lost 25 per cent of my body strength during the time I was bedridden. I remember asking, 'What happens next?', and then, 'What's happened so far?' If someone had told me I'd been in hospital for a year, I'd have believed them. I had no idea of time, and my body clock was all over the place. Once I phoned Sarah thinking it was about 10 a.m. She was normally at my bedside by that time, so I picked up my mobile and rang her. 'Can you come now, babe?' I asked.

'John, it's 3 a.m.,' she said. 'Let's both get some sleep. I'll be with you first thing.'

There wasn't one defining moment when I actually came round and rejoined the world. It was gradual and erratic, and my mind played tricks.

Looking back, I vaguely remember my dad telling me about Lance Armstrong, saying he had beaten the same thing as me. I think that is one of my first clear memories. I remember lots of other things, too, things that didn't actually happen then but were kicking around my head.

The days were long, and my mind was starting to get more active. I can't remember exactly when certain memories came to me, but I presume it was around this time, when I was starting to wake up and beginning to take stock of my life and what had happened.

They were real memories, not fantasies, so I can't be sure I relived them in all this detail in hospital, or whether my old memories caught up with my hospital memories as I wrote this down. Here goes. Welcome to the inside of my sore head. I will attempt to show you what it was like in there.

I can smell the chemicals on the hospital sheet as I pull it over my face. It's warm in my bed, and I want to sleep.

I am roasting hot now, lying by the pool in Marbella. 'I'm going to get a cold beer, babe.'

Sarah smiles. I stand up and cast a huge shadow over her. I feel like a giant. It is the summer of 2006. I am a star player for Celtic, a striker who has knocked in more than a hundred goals in five years.

I am on the pitch at Anfield now. It's a pitch I dreamed of playing on as a small boy, when Liverpool was my favourite team. I never imagined I'd be a Celtic striker, facing Liverpool in the UEFA Cup. I look at my diary and see I am dreaming of 20 March 2003, a date I will never forget.

The Kop is swaying spectacularly. There are 45,000 fans in the crowd. Squint and they are a giant flamenco dancer, swirling her red-and-white skirt and clicking her heels in a noisy, passionate display. I catch my breath when I think of the footballing gods who have trodden this pitch before me, Big John, a lad from a council estate in Swansea. It is unreal, a dream come true.

We are not expected to beat Liverpool on their home turf, but so what? Why not? I see Emile Heskey, Michael Owen, Jamie Carragher, Dietmar Hamann and Steven Gerrard. I puff out my chest.

I must do something special today. My mam and dad are in the crowd. I remember how delighted I was when they bought me a Liverpool kit when I was eight years old. It must have cost them a fortune. I want to repay them, and I want them to feel proud. That feeling intensifies when Alan Thompson puts us ahead.

The Kop drowns out our 3,000 or so visiting fans, but I can smell success. I want us to win so badly. We need another goal, and I am going to get it.

Our keeper Rab Douglas has delivered a long ball and I am going to collect it. I am fouled by Sami Hyypiä. The ref doesn't see it. I snort like a raging bull. My blood is up. I want the best revenge there is. I want a goal. I am going to get a goal.

I do a quick one-two with Henrik Larsson. When the ball comes back to me, I drop my shoulder and touch the ball past Dietmar Hamann.

It's the 82nd minute and the ball is rolling perfectly for me now, but the net is thirty yards away at least. There is red all around. Red shirts. Red scarves. Red faces. Red mist in my eyes.

I strike the ball as hard as I can. It flies into the top corner. I am flying too. I am as light as the strings on the net, and I am floating in the air. It is the best goal I have scored, ever. Celtic are through to the semi-final of a major European competition for the first time in years. I am breathless.

I am back in the sun in Marbella, panting with the heat. 'I'll be back in a minute, Sarah. Just going to cool down, just going to grab a beer.'

I am switching on Sky Sports in the apartment. I read the headlines along the bottom of the screen. As I do so, I open the fridge and an icy blast of air hits me in the face. 'Celtic has agreed a fee with West Brom for John Hartson . . .'

My throat closes over. I sway a little and clutch the fridge to steady myself. I have been sold. I am unwanted property, surplus to requirements at Celtic. Nobody has even bothered to warn me.

I brood and worry and think and fret for days, and eventually Gordon Strachan calls me. He is on holiday in Barbados. 'I thought I'd give you a couple of days to calm down, Big Man.'

'I'm OK,' I say. 'I'm calm, it's no problem.'

I hear myself and I think I am speaking the truth.

I put the phone down and remember the good times. I remember that goal at Anfield and have an intense recollection of that feeling of euphoria. That can never be taken from me. I remember my skin prickling with pride, every muscle in my body aching and the rush of blood pumping the most incredible lightning bolts of sheer joy through my brain. I can feel my brain throbbing.

I have had an amazing time at Celtic, but my time is up. I can feel the ground shifting. My football has suffered because of my personal life, the divorce. I can't deny it. I actually feel a small tremor of relief as I stretch out on my sun bed. I can move closer to my kids. Thank God for that. No more flights just to pick them up from school. Less guilt.

'You know what, Sarah, Gordon is 1,000 per cent right,' I am saying. 'I have to get down to the Midlands, make a fresh start at West Brom. The timing is right.'

'I'll be with you,' Sarah says. 'Whatever happens, I'll be with you.'

I can hear her saying it in her gorgeous Scottish accent, just like she is standing beside me, and then I actually feel the warmth of her breath on my cheek.

'I'm here, John,' she says. I open my eyes, and she is holding her face above mine as I lie in my hospital bed. 'I'm here.'

'That's good,' I muttered. 'It's good to see you.' It really was. I always know where I am with Sarah.

I listened to Sarah chatting about Lina and nursery school and all the plans for the new baby, but I found it difficult to concentrate and my mind kept wandering.

The card that Arsène Wenger and the Arsenal lads had sent caught my eye. It was propped up on the trolley next to my bed, and it immediately triggered happy memories of me pulling on an Arsenal football shirt. I shut my eyes and the shirt became a Wales one and then a Celtic one. I remembered scoring lots of goals in my green-and-white Hoops shirt. I saw my best ones in slow motion, as if they were being played on a big screen in my head. I hammered home two goals against Livingston at Parkhead. The atmosphere was electrifying. I could still sense it, and my heart raced. Henrik scored a hat-trick and we won 5–1, helping us win the SPL title. It was my first and best season at Celtic, my first title win, and best of all I proved myself as one of the 'Bhoys'. I don't know if I was remembering the actual night itself or remembering my Celtic tribute night earlier that year, when those goals were replayed on a giant screen. I've no idea.

Another time I opened my eyes in a panic and immediately tried to lift myself off the bed. I was too weak to move, and I remembered saying to the doctor, 'Do you mind undoing my bootlaces?' I remembered he looked alarmed.

'Are you serious, Big Man? You just scored. You just played 90 minutes.'

I was recalling playing for Celtic in the 2002–03 season. The doctor was Roddy Macdonald, the Celtic team doctor. My back had been playing up, and I couldn't bend far enough to take off my own boots. I had a ruptured disc, but it was a routine football injury from years of wear and tear, and I played on. My dad travelled up from Wales to watch me play against Rangers in a Premiership match. We were fresh from our victory over Boavista when we won our first European final place in 33 years. Now, with my dad in the crowd, we beat Rangers 1–2, and I scored.

'Well done, son!' my dad said afterwards. 'That was a great goal, son.'

I was subbed after 75 minutes, and my back was niggling. My dad and I had a couple of beers to celebrate the victory, but when I woke up the next morning I couldn't move. I felt like my back had been nailed to the mattress.

Reliving this from a hospital bed made me feel very uncomfortable. Then, like now, I wanted to jump out of bed and spring into my day, but it was impossible. I tried to move, but the pain was intense, like someone was sticking a needle into a nerve in my spine and twisting it every time I tried to turn. Remembering that pain reminded me of my painful headaches.

I touched my head and felt the bandages wrapped around my skull. 'You've had a few operations,' Sarah told me. 'They've all been very successful. You are on the road to recovery.'

My bad back had been cured by an operation. A disc in my spine had 'burst' and was leaking. I remembered waking up on a private ward just like this one, except it was the Ross Hall Hospital in Glasgow. That was six years ago. Now I'd had a leak in my brain fixed.

'Your body's like a patchwork quilt, John,' Sarah smiled. 'But it's all sewn up now. It's time for chemo.'

I remember doctors and nurses and a physiotherapist visiting me. A stream of people examined me, chatted to me and then walked away. I hated feeling incapacitated. It was the worst feeling in the world. I was like a prisoner in that bed, and I didn't like it one bit. Every time someone walked away I wanted to jump up and walk out the door behind them, but I had no energy in my body.

My dad always made sure he was there if I needed him. He helped to take me to the toilet, and every morning he put ten pounds on my bedside locker so I could buy a newspaper. Just knowing he was looking out for me was a comfort, although I still never felt at ease in hospital.

I looked at my dad and remembered rooting in his coat pockets when I was about five years old, watching him play up front in a football match for Afan Lido. Once I found his false teeth wrapped in a tissue, and I took them out and played with them in the sand.

I pictured myself sitting on his shoulders while he played cards with his friends, and then I remembered him tying the laces on my football boots, time and time again. He was massive in my career. The full force of his power hit me as I lay there, and each time I looked at him he went up in my estimation.

I looked at my dad's huge hands as he pulled the tenner from his wallet one morning. He's a man amongst men, my dad, a grafter, a rock. 'My hand is a baby's hand compared to yours,' I thought. While other people had fallen to bits, my dad had got stronger, Sarah said. He had stood tall and given updates for the 50 or 60 people who streamed into the waiting room. He had slept in the corridor and abandoned his business so he could be by my side. Sarah had told me this, and I was very moved. I was very lucky to have such support.

Sarah was a source of great strength too. She asked question after question to the point where the medical staff must have thought she was a nightmare, but I felt blessed to have her on my side. She and my dad had both been my eyes and ears when I was too ill to know what was happening, and I still needed them to help me through this final stage. I longed to go home with them, but I knew I still had work to do.

One day the physio gave me elastic bands to stretch over my head to strengthen my arms, and I grasped them like they were keys to unlock a prison cell.

I willingly did my exercises and did exactly as I was told. 'There's a first!' Sarah joked. I managed a smile, but I felt uncomfortable. I was used to being so active, and I didn't feel I belonged here.

Soon the physio led me over to a Zimmer frame beside the bed. Sarah encouraged me. 'I know you can do it, John. The stronger you get, the quicker you'll get home.' She couldn't have said anything better. I put one foot in front of the other, and I did it again, then again, and again.

Thursday, 30 July 2009

Sarah had been on the phone. She was up at the hospital and John had taken four steps on the Zimmer frame. That was what Mamgu used to use in her latter days, when she couldn't walk, and now John was kind of learning to walk again on one. How uncanny? It couldn't have been doing anything for John's dignity and pride when you think about it, love him xx.

JOHN

I began to remember grainy snapshots of things that had happened over the last few weeks. I remembered asking to see Bec and Joni and crying in front of them, and I remembered crying when Frances came in, because I was so relieved she was there to support Sarah. I also had a distant memory of thinking, 'I'm not going to make it though the night, I'm not going to see my next child born,' but then having a sort of sixth sense that really I would make it, even though it was going to be very tough.

When Sarah told me all about the visitors I'd had, the media coverage and the thousands of cards and messages of support I'd received, I couldn't believe it.

My dad told me about the hundreds of phone calls and messages he'd had too, some from well-known mates of mine. I couldn't believe the list: Vinnie Jones, Ian Woosnam, Joe Calzaghe, Bradley Walsh, Tony Thorpe, Alan Stubbs, Jimmy Tarbuck, John Toshack, Ryan Giggs, Alex McLeish . . . It touched my heart to think all those busy people had taken the time and trouble to get in touch. Mickey Thomas had sent me a copy of Lance Armstrong's autobiography to inspire me in my recovery. Martin O'Neill, whose wife, Geraldine, had had cancer, told me, 'I know what you're going through.' He had been so instrumental in my career, and it meant so much to know he was rooting for me. Harry Redknapp wrote, 'I love you to pieces, you've got to get through this.'

Gordon Strachan had been in touch with my dad throughout, and he sent lots of messages. When he found out I'd gone down to 14 stone, he joked, 'If you'd have lost all this weight before, I'd have signed you again . . .' I laughed. Moments like that helped me get though the long, boring days in hospital.

Mam came in the evenings and brought me all the things she knew I liked, like tuna-and-mayo sandwiches, Quavers and sweets. We watched *Coronation Street* or *EastEnders* together, and it felt almost normal. She's a very emotional person, but she never broke down in front of me. It was a real comfort to have her beside me.

After a couple of days I started asking more questions, and I asked Sarah to fill me in with more details. She talked me though the journey so far, and I listened in a sort of horrified amazement.

'And then the machine started bleeping and I realised you had stopped breathing . . .'

'Your dad's feet went from under him . . .'

'It was touch and go whether you'd make it to the Morriston for the brain op . . .'

The detail astonished me. I felt terrible for the worry I'd put everyone through. 'What now?' I asked.

'Another day in here, then it's back to the Singleton for chemo. You'll have four weeks of intensive chemo, administered through a drip, with two weeks off in between each five-day course. With a bit of luck, they'll discharge you after the first course – and they're going to let you go out for a day trip when you've managed a few more paces on the Zimmer.'

I was desperate to get out of hospital. All the staff were fantastic, but I never felt relaxed there. I felt nervous and vulnerable. I wanted to run down the corridor and escape in my car, but, of course, it wasn't like that. When I was allowed out for my day trip, I staggered out on a Zimmer frame feeling like an old man.

I felt envious of other people, jumping into their cars. They were probably going to Tesco's or picking the kids up from school. Normal stuff, but stuff I couldn't take for granted any more.

'Look what you've done!' Dad said as I shuffled out into the warm sunshine, gripping the Zimmer. It was great to feel fresh air on my face again, but I was a long way from celebrating.

I caught a look at myself in a car mirror and was shocked by what I saw. My skin was translucent, my eyes were sunk deep into my bald white head and my tracksuit looked several sizes too big on me. I'd lost five stone in a month and weighed just fourteen stone. I looked like an Aids victim or a shrivelled alcoholic. I hardly recognised myself, but other people did.

Dad had picked me up in his van, which has the name of his company – Hartson Fire – emblazoned in red lettering down the side. I wondered why he hadn't brought the car instead, as I didn't want to be recognised by anybody, but I didn't complain.

Every time we pulled up at traffic lights, people were staring at me. I wasn't allowed in the sun and I had brought a woollen hat, so I put it on and pulled it down as far as I could without covering my eyes. The most important thing was that I was out of hospital, but nevertheless I didn't want to put on a freak show.

When we reached the Mumbles, I had to steel myself to get out of the van and stagger a few yards. 'Well done! Look what you've achieved, John!' Dad was so proud, so relieved.

I lay down on the grass and just pulled a blanket over my head. Lina was there. I remember her inquisitive little face. She didn't know what to make of me. She hadn't seen her daddy for weeks and weeks, and he'd had a dramatic change in appearance. She clung to Sarah and eyed me cautiously, and then jumped all over my head. It hurt, but I pulled her onto my chest. It was a joy to see her again. I had missed her so much.

My dad bought me a Joe's chocolate-chip ice cream. The Mumbles is famous for them, and normally I'd have to stop myself eating two. Now I could barely hold the cornet to my lips, let alone eat it. Next Dad appeared with a bag of chips and tried to get me to eat them instead. 'Come on, John, we don't want you wasting away! Just have a couple!' I couldn't eat a single one.

I lay back down, looked at the clouds and breathed deeply. The grass and daisies had a powerful, sweet smell and a breeze was carrying Lina's babbles and giggles to my ears.

The trip had reminded me that there was life outside the hospital walls, and I was grateful for that. But I knew I had a very long way to go to get back to my old self. My chemo hadn't even started yet, and I wondered how the hell I would get through it. I didn't know a thing about chemo. Sarah had told me it would be given to me through a drip, but I really didn't know what to expect.

Returning to the hospital later that afternoon was depressing, even though the trip had shown me I wasn't yet capable of fending for myself.

'How much longer do I have to stay in here?' I asked Sarah. She was pulling the sheets up around me, fussing around me as best she could with Lina swinging on her hip. I was back in a hospital bed, and I didn't like it one bit. 'I've tasted freedom now,' I said, attempting a joke but sounding bitter and serious. 'I want to come home with you and Lina.'

Sunday, 2 August 2009

John was transferred from Morriston to Singleton. We were overjoyed. He would begin an intense course of chemotherapy at the Singleton over the next few days and take it from there. Sarah gave him a nice shower in his private room, and we all told him how much we'd continue to support and visit him daily, until he was well enough to come out.

JOHN

Now I was in a private room on the top floor of the Singleton Hospital. I had practically no recollection of being treated there before, but the staff all seemed to know me. The nurses gave me a bit of VIP treatment and said they thought I'd be more comfortable up in a room of my own rather than on a ward.

People were questioning why I was being treated on the NHS, and the simple reason was that it offered the best possible care in the vicinity. Peter Lawwell, the Celtic chairman, had phoned my dad, offering to pay for me to be cared for at the private Sancta Maria Hospital. It's a fabulous place, but it didn't offer radiotherapy and I would have had to travel back and forth during that stage of my treatment, which wasn't a good idea.

Besides, I was extremely well cared for at the Singleton, just as I had been at the Morriston. I had a large, bright room with a big TV, and Kath, my physiotherapist, was brilliant.

'We can't discharge you until you get a bit stronger and a bit steadier on your feet,' she explained. 'Twenty-five per cent of your body strength is a lot to lose.'

'I feel OK, though; I reckon I could manage with the Zimmer,' I said to Kath hopefully one morning. 'Perhaps I could come in as a day patient for all of the chemo?'

Sarah stepped in, cutting to the chase as usual. She shook her head. 'John, they can't discharge you until they can be sure you're not going to fall over and split your head on the pavement.'

I looked at her and my eyes fell to her stomach. She had a neat but very visible bump now, and with Lina now toddling around I suddenly realised how much Sarah had on her plate. There was no way I wanted to be an extra burden to her, however desperate I was to get out of hospital.

I was having physio three or four times a week to help rebuild my muscle and strength, and I worked my backside off to do everything Kath asked of me. 'I thought I'd finished with daily training,' I joked whenever she appeared, but I did my exercises willingly and to the letter. I had one eye on the door most of the time, willing the day to come when I could walk back out of it unaided, but I poured my energy into getting stronger.

Tuesday, 4 August

So Chemotherapy Begins

My dad arrived at the hospital nice and early in readiness for the chemo to begin.

I knew my dad was the best person to accompany John through anything. Something stuck in my mind that Mam had said to me. We were talking a few days previously about how wonderful my dad had been – he was John's pillar – the footprints in the sand – whichever way you wanted to describe it. Anyway, I was saying how my dad was practically there 24/7 and he didn't care for his business and he didn't leave John's side. If he wasn't in John's room he was in the waiting room outside and only ever slipped home when John was fast asleep. My mam said that my dad had told her: 'I will not leave the hospital until John can walk out with me.' That was so touching, and he meant it.

John began his chemotherapy at 11.45 a.m. today. Initially we were under the impression that the chemo would take three hours to go from the drip into the bloodstream, but we were told that in fact he was having three different kinds of chemo and it would actually take four to five hours. How intense must that be! Poor John.

My dad said that John got very emotional just as the treatment was beginning. I suppose the build-up was a lot to take. We'd been talking about having chemo for over a week now and all of a sudden it was here.

Prepare to be ill!

Everyone had said how ill John was going to be. I know how bad a hangover is the day after a good night out, but these were deadly chemicals running though your bloodstream, killing off all the bad cells but wiping out the good, too. Just the thought of it was enough to make you ill.

We all had to remain positive and remember John *needed* this chemo to get well – there was no way around it. 'Maybe he won't be that ill,' we kept saying to one another. 'Not everyone is ill with it,' I'd say.

I phoned my dad at teatime and he said John was sitting up, feeling fine and eating sponge and custard. We were saying that maybe we had been right and he wouldn't be that ill – I mean, the chemo is instant, and it was in his bloodstream, working instantly. The doctors had said that everyone responds differently. It was early days, and we'd have to see.

JOHN

Chemotherapy. I'd heard the word a million times but never in a million years thought I would actually be having it. I had virtually no experience of cancer. I knew two other footballers who had survived testicular cancer: Alan Stubbs, who played for Everton, and Rangers' Craig Moore. But I'd never lost anyone close to me, and I knew nothing about how chemo worked.

I soon learned that there are hundreds of types of chemo drugs, and everybody's chemo is different depending on things like your height and weight and what parts of the body it needs to target.

A nurse explained that I would have three types of chemo to begin with, then a course of bleomycin, a particularly potent type of chemo used to blast away testicular cancer. It is so powerful it can damage the lungs, and I remember thinking: 'All that training, all that running: it's payback time. My lungs are powerful enough to take this. They're as strong as anything.'

'Bleomycin is a powder that dissolves to form a colourless liquid,' the nurse explained. 'As with all of your chemo, you'll receive it via a drip into your Hickman line.' I nodded obediently.

I'd had the Hickman line fitted under local anaesthetic. I was having so much chemo the doctors said that was the best way to get it into me; otherwise, if they had to find a vein each time I'd be like a pincushion and they may run out of veins to use. The line was basically a plastic tube that went directly into my chest. It felt very intrusive. I could feel it twisting and turning, fat pulling on muscle, but in the big scheme of things it was nothing. Just another inconvenience I had to put up with to get this cancer beaten.

The nurse went on to list the possible side effects of my chemo. Normally I would glaze over when someone launched into a long explanation, but on this occasion I listened attentively, even though the list went on and on. The hair loss, sickness and extreme tiredness I already knew about. It didn't bother me in the slightest that I would lose my hair, because I was pretty well bald in any case – and who cared about eyebrows and chest hair? I couldn't have cared less. Sickness and tiredness I accepted as just par for the course. You were bound to throw up and feel knackered after being pumped full of toxic chemicals, weren't you?

But other possible side effects were news to me: fever, shivering, bleeding gums, mouth ulcers, diarrhoea, memory problems, nose bleeds, breathing difficulties – the list just went on and on.

'Bring it on,' I said. 'What will be will be.'

I was given a record card listing my chemo schedule. I would have three bags a day for five days, then a fortnight off. The pattern would repeat for three months, and in total I would have sixty-seven bags of chemo. I'd never heard of anyone having so much, and it brought it home to me just how bad the cancer was.

I felt a bit wobbly when I went into the chemo ward for the first session. I was more mentally alert than I had been in weeks, and I think the enormity of what I had been through, and what I still had to go through, was only just starting to hit me. A lovely nurse called Hannah had a chat with me, and Kerry, who was in charge of chemo, couldn't have done more. They explained that it would probably take from 9 a.m. to 3 p.m. to get all the chemo in me. All I had to do was sit there and take it.

My dad kept me company that first day while Sarah looked after Lina. It must have been so boring for him, but he chatted to me about anything and everything. I remember he told me Vic was going to do the Kilvey Hill cement run for charity. It's a mile-long race and women have to carry 25 kg on their back.

'I told her it's tough – she'll have to do quite a bit of training,' Dad said.

'She'll do it, Dad. She's a tough one, our Vic. She's a fighter, like me.'

Dad smiled. 'That's my boy!' he said. 'That's the sort of talk I want to hear!'

I felt like crying, and I felt absolutely no shame in crying in front of my dad, but I stopped myself. My dad had never broken down in front of me. He remained cheerful and positive and resilient, and when I looked at him that day I didn't want to burden him any more.

Having chemo was a turning point: that was the way to look at it. The drugs were killing my cancer. The chemicals were in charge now, not the cancer cells. I was going to feel worse before I got better, but I was getting better. There was no need for tears any more.

Later, after the last drop of chemo had drained from the last bag into my bloodstream and I was back on the ward, Mam arrived.

'I've brought you some M&S sponge and custard. I know it's your favourite,' she said, flicking through the TV channels and settling herself in the chair beside me. Just like my dad, she was putting on a great show of strength.

'Thanks, Mam. With a bit of luck I won't lose my appetite. This is delicious.'

The next day I started leafing through Lance Armstrong's

autobiography while I had my chemo. Someone had also printed off the message he'd left for me on Twitter. It was dated 15 July – the day after I stopped breathing. 'My thoughts go out to John Hartson,' he wrote. 'Live strong, John! We're pulling for you! Folks, hold him in your thoughts and prayers please.'

I felt inspired by the great man. I read that he had been diagnosed with testicular cancer in 1996. That was a long, long time ago. It was when I was playing for Arsenal and, to be honest, I was totally oblivious to his story at the time.

Now I wanted to know everything about him. His cancer spread to his lungs and brain, just like mine, but he'd beaten it and gone on to win the Tour de France seven times in a row, from 1999 to 2005. I wanted to be another success story, I really did.

Lance wrote about how he wanted more and more chemo to really blast the cancer out of him, to the point where he was practically begging for more. I sort of understood where he was coming from. I didn't wish any more chemo upon myself – six hours a day was quite enough – but I welcomed it into my body. As it dripped through the Hickman line I knew it was healing me, even if it was going to make me sick at the same time.

I settled into my new routine quickly. Each day I was given chemo in the same private room. I switched my mobile off, had a bit of banter with the nurses, and usually my dad and Sarah took it in turns to sit with me. I didn't really feel like chatting, but it was comforting having someone with me.

I only managed to read a few pages at a time, because I found it hard to concentrate, and eventually I decided to read Lance's book properly when I was out of hospital. It was probably a bit too much to take in at that stage, and my dad was concerned it might upset me. I think he was right.

I slept sometimes, but each time a bag emptied it beeped and woke me up. After the beep there came a kind of hiss as the last drop of fluid and air was sucked out of the bag. I'll never forget those sounds. They ruled my life for five long days that week, and I knew they would rule my life for another few months to come.

CHAPTER TWELVE

Going home

'Good luck, John.'

First one nurse said it, then another. Before I knew it, it felt like the whole hospital was wishing me luck.

'Go on, Big John!'

'Get well soon, Johnny boy!'

I was stepping out into fresh morning air, and I wasn't going back. I still had the Zimmer for support, but when I stood on the hospital steps and looked out into the world, I felt I could run a marathon. It was one of the best moments of my life.

Mam and Dad drove me home, where Sarah was waiting for me with Lina. It was 11 August, and I hadn't seen my house for over a month. I felt exhilarated, but I was exhausted, too. The chemo had started to take its toll. My appetite had dropped away over the past week, and I had a permanent feeling of nausea and sickness in my stomach. Most of all, I felt an overwhelming tiredness.

Our driveway is on a slight slope, and it was an effort just to reach the top of it and step in through the front door. I drank in the familiar sights in the hall: a vase of flowers, my Caterpillar trainers on the rack by the door, a tiny pink coat. Ordinary, everyday objects, but things I hadn't seen for weeks and weeks. It felt like a year.

It's an unusual set-up in our house. It's built on three storeys, and you enter on the middle floor and go downstairs to the kitchen and family room. Sarah rushed upstairs to greet me, with Lina in her arms. I buried my head between my two beautiful girls, holding them tight, letting their warmth and curls smother me.

The house was filled with a delicious smell of garlic, tomatoes, beef and herbs, and I could hear Bec and Joni saying, 'Daddy! It's Dad!'

'I've done a spaghetti bolognese; I know it's one of your favourites,' Sarah said.

I looked at the twisted staircase leading down to the ground floor and took in the sturdy banister to attached the wall. A Macmillan nurse had visited me in hospital, offering to help kit out our house to make it easier for me to get around while I was still weak.

'No, no,' I'd insisted. 'We don't need anything. We've got banisters and all that. I'll manage.' I think I might have said that anyway. I didn't want a charity spending its money on me; it didn't seem right. Besides, I didn't want to feel disabled. I'd had enough of that in hospital, and I'd left that behind.

Now, looking at the stairs, I was thankful we really did have a banister, because I was going to have to grip it hard to haul myself down the mountain pass my stairs had suddenly become.

'John!'

'Daddy!'

'Welcome home! It's great to have you back!'

The reception I received made the huge effort worth it. I'd only taken about 20 paces from the car to the kitchen and I was wiped out, but my family gave me a welcome home as if I'd just come back from Afghanistan.

I ate a small bowl of food and sat back with a duvet over my feet in my favourite beige suede chair in the corner of the family room, watching my world go around. I was home at last. I'd made it back.

That night, Sarah and I just held each other. It was too early for words. We just enjoyed being back together, with Lina sleeping in her cot and Sarah's bump pushing against her jeans.

There was still a long way to go. I'd only ticked off 15 bags of chemo on my card. That left 52 more bags to go. Doctors would keep testing my blood to see if the chemo had done its job, to see if the 191,000 cancer markers in my blood had been tackled. I was still shocked every time I thought of that huge number, even though it was burned into my brain.

After the chemo was finished, my testicle would be removed and my brain and lungs would have to be scanned again. I might need more operations if the tumours persisted.

On my second day back home, I managed to ditch the Zimmer and shuffle round the kitchen using our breakfast bar, which is like a central island, for support. I didn't feel ill, just very tired, and I told Sarah I felt optimistic about the chemo. I was sure it was working. After three or four days I got rid of the Zimmer completely, which made me feel better still.

After a week or so I started sleeping for hours and hours every afternoon, but I woke up still feeling wiped out. Lifting Lina completely shattered me. One morning I carried her upstairs and had to shout to Sarah, 'Take the baby, quick – I'm going to drop her.' After that I didn't even trust myself with a glass of water, let alone our daughter.

I normally love my food and Sarah cooked fantastic meals. She made homemade chips and juicy steaks, but I had completely lost my appetite and I'd push them round my plate. I knew I'd get weak if I didn't eat, so sometimes I'd force down a ham sandwich or a bit of pizza if I really hadn't eaten, but it just came back up. The same thing happened with milk. I was told to drink it to help keep mouth ulcers at bay, as they can be really irritating and can set you back, but I gagged on the milk and suffered with horrible ulcers.

Once, my mam and dad were driving me home from hospital after a chemo session when a terrible wave of sickness came over me. Mam had brought me a lunch of Lucozade and egg sandwiches – normally favourites of mine – and I'd managed a bit. We stopped at some traffic lights and I had to wind down the window to be sick. I threw up violently three more times on the way home.

I started to suffer from terrible diarrhoea, too. My clothes were hanging off me, and as the weeks went on I lost all of my hair, my eyebrows and my eyelashes. I looked a wreck, and my life just revolved around hospital visits, blood tests and lying low at home.

I had to keep telling myself over and over, 'John, you're going to survive this. You are not going to die.' Sarah told me the same thing.

'It's tough right now, but it'll get better soon,' she said. 'You're beating it.'

After a few weeks, we got our first positive news in ages. My blood markers had fallen dramatically, from the hundreds of thousands to 57. It was what we had expected and hoped for, but it was still a massive relief when Dr Bertelli read the results to us. He explained that the drop is often quite dramatic to begin with and then slows down, but all the signs were good. I was responding to the chemo very well indeed.

'Shall we take the kids to Legoland?' I said to Sarah. 'If I hadn't been ill, we would have taken them away somewhere over the summer. I want to make it up to them.'

'I don't know, John,' Sarah replied. 'You're still very weak, and I'm pregnant. Are you sure it's a good idea?'

I was adamant, and Sarah dutifully booked us a stay at the Copthorne in Windsor for a couple of days before my next chemo cycle. Bec and Joni were delighted, and little Lina was thrilled to be setting off on an adventure.

Sarah has since told me that she had her heart in her mouth right from the start, but she said nothing. She knew it was empowering for me to try to do something normal and active, to prove to myself that life was getting back to how it used to be.

We'd only been inside the park for ten minutes when I had to cling onto the railings for support. 'You go on, Sarah,' I said. I tried to put on a brave face, but inside I felt absolutely terrible. Sarah had been right. This was a disastrous idea.

I looked at her with her growing bump and felt awful. Bec and Joni were asking to go on the big roller coasters and, of course, Sarah wasn't allowed to go on. 'I'll go on with you later,' I called after them.

'John, you can't,' Sarah hissed. 'You've just had major brain surgery.'

Lina started screaming in her buggy, pushing against the straps and demanding to get out. I gritted my teeth and put one step in front of the other like my life depended on it. 'Why don't we all go on the River Splash Rapids?'

'Yay!' Bec and Joni cheered.

'I'll wait on the side with Lina; it's too big for her,' Sarah said, at which point Lina started wailing like a banshee.

We managed one or two more rides before we staggered back to the hotel. I couldn't even go for a swim with the kids, because of the Hickman line in my chest.

I felt like apologising to them, but I looked at my family and felt a surge of love. Lina was sitting contentedly in her high chair, eating pasta shapes. Bec and Joni were chatting about their favourite models in the miniature Lego cities. They had made the most of our trip, and their innocence touched my heart. When I was a kid my parents never burdened me with adult worries, and I wasn't going to spoil the moment by reminding my kids their dad was sick. I'd make it up to them when I was truly better.

A few weeks later, I suggested another trip – this time up to Scotland.

'John, you're irrepressible!' Sarah said.

'I know, that's why you love me,' I winked.

I was heading towards the end of my chemo, and even though I was still very tired and my appetite was poor, I seemed to have got over the worst of the sickness and diarrhoea. I was fed up of being stuck in the house, and I thought it would be nice to visit Sarah's parents in Fort William. I wanted to thank them for looking after Lina and for all their support, and I thought it would give Sarah a boost, too, as she hadn't been to Scotland for months.

My own parents thought it was too early for me to fly, but my mind was made up. It made me feel stronger to get back out into the real world, and thankfully this trip turned out to be a good one.

I struggled during the flight, I have to admit. I felt very tired and weak. I had had bleomycin by now, and it gave me a few palpitations and chest pains, which I'd been warned could happen as the chemical attacked the tumours in my lungs. I had to take a deep breath just to talk.

Sarah was a trouper. She held my hand tight and took me to an old haunt of ours, a cafe in Fort William that specialises in spit roasts. I have always really loved their meat rolls, and even though my appetite was nowhere near normal, I found myself tucking in to not one but two delicious pork rolls. It was the most I'd eaten in ages.

I felt the best I had since leaving hospital. Sarah looked fairly relaxed too and went for a stroll around the shops, although she admitted to me much later that she had a 'moment' when she completely lost it. A shop assistant simply asked her, 'How is John?' and she burst into tears.

'I had a total meltdown; I've no idea where it came from,' she told me later. 'I ran to the toilets and sobbed my heart out.' On the day itself, I had no idea.

After lunch, we sat on a bench in a garden near Sarah's parents' house. From there I could see the stunning Scottish mountaintops, with Ben Nevis shimmering in a purple-and-amber haze in the distance. It looked magnificent, and I gazed at it longingly. I'd spent weeks and weeks staring at sterile white walls and bags of drugs, and breathing in that cloying hospital air. Now I was filling my lungs with fresh mountain air and imagining what it would be like to conquer Britain's biggest mountain.

It looked like it was for ever and a day away from me, but in that moment I made a decision: I was going to climb it.

'I'm going up there,' I told Sarah.

Her eyes widened. 'John, you need to take one step at a time . . .'

'Not today!' I reassured her. 'I'll have trouble getting up off this bench today. But one day I'll get up that mountain. One day, when I have beaten this thing, I will stand on top of Ben Nevis and say: "I survived." That's a promise.' I had no idea if it would take me a year or a decade. Only one thing was certain – I was climbing it.

I finished my chemo in October. I can't say I felt any different after the last bag had drained into me than I had after the 66 bags that went before it.

I was relieved that stage of my treatment was over, because I was bored rigid with chemo, but it was too early for celebrations. I had no idea whether it had completed its work or whether I'd need more treatment. It was a waiting game now. I was to have another CAT scan in a few weeks, and my blood markers would be tested again.

In the meantime, Sarah and I had a much better type of scan on our minds – her 20-week antenatal scan, which would tell us the sex of our new baby.

We must have looked like a pretty odd couple when we turned up at the maternity clinic. I was as bald as a coot, my skin was the colour of the pavement and I was shuffling along like an old man, while Sarah was blossoming and glowing and bouncing along with roses in her cheeks, looking more gorgeous than ever. Still, it was fantastic to be going into hospital for something positive for once.

I felt very proud of Sarah when she lay back on the bed waiting for the radiographer to show us the baby. You would never have guessed at the hell she'd been dragged through, she simply looked radiant.

Sarah wanted another girl, and I really hoped she would get her wish. It's what I wanted, too. It somehow felt right for Lina to get a sister and for Joni to be my only boy.

'I'm pleased to tell you that's a little baby girl you are carrying,' the radiographer smiled. We both burst out laughing and tears sprang from Sarah's eyes. It was such a relief, such a pleasure.

'How lucky are we?' she said.

'You deserved some good news, Sarah. Well done.' I kissed her on the forehead. 'I'll be there for you when you have the baby, don't worry about that,' I told her.

I had started giving a few interviews by this stage, and whenever journalists asked me the questions 'did you think you were going to die?' or 'do you think you are going to beat this?' I always categorically said, 'Yes.' My stock answer had been: 'Yes, I'm confident my blood markers will return to normal, and after a few more bits of surgery I will be on the road to a full recovery.' 'I am going to live to see my baby born,' became my new line now.

Sarah was always by my side, so she heard me say this over and over again to journalists. In private, I said the same thing to her. Without ever really discussing any sort of coping strategy, we had both instinctively adopted the same positive attitude to my cancer. We both put on a brave face, refused to discuss worst-case scenarios and focused completely and utterly on my full recovery. 'I couldn't possibly walk round thinking I was on borrowed time,' I told one reporter. 'That would just be too horrific for words.'

Victoria had been on at me almost from the day I came out of hospital to start a charitable foundation to raise awareness of testicular cancer and help other cancer sufferers. She's a doer, and she knows I have always done my best to support different charities along the way.

It was clearly a good idea. I could stand in front of a class of first-team apprentices and tell them to check themselves regularly, and because I was one of the lads, they would listen. If someone had done that in front of me, maybe I wouldn't have ignored my lump. Victoria agreed to do the initial legwork, because I didn't have the foggiest idea how to start a foundation, and I didn't have the mental strength either just yet. My cousin Mark helped a great deal, too.

When I was alone, I had moments when I felt very low. I deeply regretted not looking after my health better, and I began to regret more than ever how much money I had gambled away. Warnings my dad had given me over the years echoed around my head. 'You won't play football for ever, John. You need to save some money, make some wise investments.'

I'd bought three apartments in Swansea in recent years, one of my better financial moves. But I still felt sick when I thought about the thousands I'd wasted and was still wasting right up until the point I was ill.

I wanted to put my house in order, make sure my kids and Sarah were well provided for. I had never felt so protective over them, yet I had never been so weak.

'I'm really sorry, Sarah,' I said one night. Lina was fast asleep, and I could hear her snuffles on the baby monitor. Bec and Joni were sleeping over too – Bec in her pink bed, Joni in his blue one. They shared a room when they stayed over and complained about it, but I told them they didn't know how lucky they were. I clung onto that remark. Despite my gambling habit, I was lucky enough to still be able to provide for my children. They had more than I'd ever had as a kid, and had never gone without. I would always make sure they were well provided for.

'It must have been a shock when you went over the accounts,' I said to Sarah. She had told me plainly and simply what she had discovered. 'I thought I could still have the odd flutter and get away with it. I'm sorry.'

Sarah was in an uncomfortable position. She looked exasperated, and under normal circumstances she'd have probably blown her stack, with very good reason. Instead, she took a deep breath and stayed very calm. That was something cancer had taught us both to do. Bickering and fighting seemed such a waste of time and energy now. Why waste precious moments of your life being cross and upset and raking up the past?

Despite all our brave and positive talk, we both knew there was a possibility I still might not survive, and we didn't want to spoil the time we shared. Cancer has killed stronger men than me. We knew that, even if we didn't mention it. In the next few weeks we'd have the big powwow with Dr Bertelli, which would tell us whether the chemo had worked. That was what mattered most.

'Look, John,' Sarah said flatly. 'I'm not going to row with you now, but this is a wake-up call. You simply have to stop gambling. You have to accept it is an addiction, and you need to stop kidding yourself it's some sort of hobby. I think when you are well enough you should go and have some proper counselling.'

I nodded sheepishly.

The last of my old cash cards had been destroyed, and Sarah was going to take total care of all our finances and transfer small amounts of pocket money into one new account that I would use when I was on my own.

'Thanks,' I said. It was a weight off my mind. I trusted Sarah implicitly. She was the one person I could really have a heart-to-heart with, and despite my faults she was on my side, supporting me and always striving to make life better for us both.

'I'd like to get married sooner rather than later,' I added. 'We've waited long enough. Let's just do it.'

Sarah was heavily pregnant by now, and she started chattering about how she'd need to get into shape after the baby, and how July next year would be perfect, just as we'd already discussed. We'd already looked at local venues and had our eye on the Vale Resort hotel in the Vale of Glamorgan, but we hadn't made any final decisions.

'That would give me a good couple of months to get myself sorted . . .'

'I meant sooner than that,' I said.

Sarah looked surprised, and then saddened. It was obvious what I was thinking, but it was unsayable. If we got bad news, I could die. Even if it wasn't bad news, I still faced several more operations, and I still might not survive.

A few days later, I went back into the Singleton to have my right testicle removed. After what I'd been through, the operation felt minor in the extreme. Sarah had asked me how I felt about the surgery and discussed the possibility of me having a prosthetic testicle, but the thought had never crossed my mind. As we'd said so many times, my body was already like a patchwork quilt. Having one ball removed was neither here nor there. I didn't consider it an affront to my manhood or anything like that. It certainly wasn't on a par with the way a woman might feel about having a breast removed. I'd simply be glad to get shot of the thing that had turned my life upside down. There was no fuss. I've worried about going to the dentist more than I did about going in for that op.

'Good riddance,' I thought before I was sedated, and when I woke up I thought, 'Thank God for that. Another hurdle jumped. Bring on the next one. Get me closer to the finishing line.'

I was left with a really big scar along the side of my groin, and I stayed in hospital for one night feeling a bit sore, but I was given a tube of cream and released the next day.

'It makes you unique,' Sarah said when I showed her the damage. 'Er, I see it's not going to stop you walking round the house naked then,' she laughed.

'No, and it won't stop me going commando-style in my kilt at the wedding either,' I teased.

We spent the day running through all the possible wedding scenarios.

Go abroad? No, I was too ill for a long flight. Bring the big wedding forward? No, Sarah was too big and it was too short notice. Gretna Green? No, we didn't have to run away!

We came to the conclusion the best solution was to have a private ceremony in the local registry office and then have a big wedding party at the Vale of Glamorgan in July, as we wanted, renewing our vows and inviting all our family and friends.

We'd keep the initial ceremony low-key, just me and Sarah. We didn't want to offend anybody, so we decided it was best to invite nobody. Sarah called the registry office to book us in, only to discover we had to have a couple of witnesses.

'Mark and Joanne?' We both said the names together. Mark is not only my cousin but also one of my closest friends. He was engaged to Joanne, and they lived three doors down from us. Both had offered unstinting support over the last few months. Before I was ill, after a few glasses of wine one night, we'd all joked that we should have a joint wedding. We knew they had already discussed a registry office ceremony, so we asked them if they'd be our witnesses and offered to be theirs at the same time. To our delight, they readily agreed, and we all swore each other to secrecy.

Sarah paid forty pounds to Neath Registry Office and booked the service for 4 December, two days after my big meeting with Dr Bertelli.

'If it's bad news, at least Sarah will be Mrs Hartson,' I thought privately. 'I don't want to leave her behind with a load of hassle because we weren't married.'

'Hopefully we'll get good news and we'll have a great double celebration,' I told Sarah.

'Course we will,' she said.

I was grateful for the distraction the wedding brought. We laughed our heads off sorting out the outfits. Sarah was 'rotund', as she put it, while I looked like my former body had been pricked with a giant needle and I'd deflated into a shrunken version of myself.

We ordered wedding rings from the same Stratford jewellers we'd bought Sarah's engagement ring from, but then found out they wouldn't be ready in time. Under normal circumstances this would have been a disaster, but we turned it into a positive and decided we would make do with some old rings and exchange our new wedding rings in front of family and friends in July.

'You know what, if that had happened before you got ill I'd have gone absolutely mental,' Sarah admitted. 'But it doesn't matter really, does it? What matters is that we're getting married.'

I nodded. We'd both changed. We'd calmed down, and trivial problems didn't bother us. Now what mattered most of all was that I lived to see my new wife deliver my new baby in March.

I had a CAT scan the week before the wedding, and my blood samples were taken to test the cancer markers. As the day of the big verdict from Dr Bertelli drew closer, I was starting to feel nervous and a bit run down. My Hickman line was still in place, and it had become infected. I had developed terrible thrush in my mouth – an after-effect of the chemo drugs – and I was dosed up with antibiotics. I told everyone that I wasn't too worried about the meeting, but really I was very worried indeed.

I thought about the worst-case scenario. What if the cancer markers were still high? What if my body hadn't been receptive and the chemo hadn't worked? I think my worry manifested itself in my physical state, and I felt rougher than I had done for weeks.

My appointment was at 3.40 p.m. on 2 December. We busied ourselves with Lina in the morning. She was walking now, and she had a habit of toddling up to me and putting her arms out for a hug. I was nervous every time she did it, because of the Hickman line, and I couldn't wait to get rid of it. I cuddled her tight nevertheless that day, and told her to be a good girl at nursery.

Sarah and I drove to the hospital in virtual silence and arrived at the waiting room outside Dr Bertelli's office at 3.39 p.m.

'I know you'll be cancer free when we have our big wedding party,' Sarah said.

We were like a couple of coiled springs. Sarah sounded breathless, and I realised I was practically holding my breath too.

'John Hartson,' a nurse called, and I grabbed Sarah's hand. As soon as I saw Dr Bertelli's face appear in the doorway, I knew it was good news. He had a big smile on his face, but I still held my breath. Dr Bertelli talks very quietly, and I didn't want to miss a thing. Sarah and I were squeezing each other's hands so tight we were practically yanking them off.

'It's really good news,' Dr Bertelli said. 'It's remarkable how your cancer markers have come down. They're almost zero – they have dropped to just two.'

I was dumbfounded. Sarah burst into tears and was trying desperately hard not to make too much of a scene, but then I started crying too, and we both started sobbing and hugging each other.

'Would you like to see your scans now?' Dr Bertelli asked.

'Yes please, thank you!' I said, and couldn't stop myself stepping forward and giving Dr Bertelli a hug too. 'Thank you, doctor.'

He showed us 'before' and 'after' scans and explained that I still had some 'masses' in my lungs and brain. They had examined my testicle when it was removed, and it also contained a 'mass' but had no live cancer cells. They expected the masses in my lungs and brain to also be cancer-free, but I would need two operations to open up my lungs and examine the lumps, and possibly more brain surgery to check out one large mass at the back of my head.

We talked about a timescale, and I asked if we could get Christmas out of the way and book the surgery for the New Year, or even after the baby arrived in March.

'We've got a lot going on,' I said gratefully to Dr Bertelli, and he nodded and smiled. I looked at Sarah and knew she was thinking the same thing as me. Thank God we had a lot going on, a lot of things that had nothing to do with cancer. Life was almost back how we wanted it. It was just two days before we were due to get married, and now it certainly would be a double celebration, and more.

We picked up Lina from nursery, collected a bottle of champagne from Tesco's and raised a glass. 'To the future!' Sarah said. 'I never doubted those results for one minute.'

I started phoning everyone I knew with the news. 'Zero – yes, zero! He said it's remarkable!' Sarah said I sounded like an excited child, but

I was cautious to add, 'Of course, it doesn't mean I'm completely out of the woods yet . . . I haven't been given the all-clear, so to speak. They don't give you the all-clear at this stage . . . you have to be all-clear for five years for that . . .'

I felt superb. I felt the all-clear was within my grasp, and the fact there was no rush to operate on my lungs or the mass in my brain filled me with confidence.

The next day, while Sarah flitted around sorting out her hair and nails and wedding outfit I had my Hickman line removed. It had been a constant reminder of my chemotherapy, and it was very satisfying to see it dumped in a bin marked 'clinical waste – dispose of by incineration'.

I suppose I should have been out having some sort of a stag drink the day before my wedding, but I was just happy to have that plastic pipe taken away, go home and be able to have my first shower in months.

I slept like a baby that night. My mind felt lighter than it had in ages. I could think clearly, and when we floated into the registry office the next day I couldn't believe my luck.

'I, Sarah Ann McManus, take you, John Hartson, to be my husband, to have and to hold from this day forward, for better or for worse, for richer, for poorer, in sickness and in health, to love and to cherish from this day forward until death do us part.'

It felt like we were actors in a film. I couldn't believe we'd actually made it this far, and this was for real.

I don't know what set us off, but it happened at the same moment. I don't think it was the word 'sickness' or even 'death'. It was just a powerful pang of love that struck us both at the same time.

Sarah looked up at me and I stared at her, incredulous at this beautiful pregnant woman in front of me, holding my hand, becoming my wife. My lip trembled and so did hers, though neither of us cried. Perhaps we'd got used to stopping ourselves from crying.

I'll never forget that moment.

Sarah had glossy ringlets in her hair and glowing skin. She looked delicate and precious, despite her huge baby bump, and I couldn't believe she had been such a powerhouse of strength. I had shrunk. I'd lost my bulk and my power and I was getting used to being an average 14-st. man. Sarah had got bigger with our baby growing inside her, and her strength had grown, too.

After the service, we piled into a limousine with Mark and Joanne and went to a rooftop restaurant in Swansea. Nobody there knew we'd just got married. We had a slap-up meal and a glass of champagne, and Sarah said she was glad to be able to sit down and have a rest. Her ankles were swollen and she had to keep going to the ladies, and we were both wiped out with tiredness at the end of the day, but we had no regrets. So many parts of my life had been played out in public, and it was good to have kept this day private.

'Happy?' I asked Sarah.

'Very,' she replied.

In that moment, that was all that mattered.

Inevitably, when word got out that we'd got married 'in secret' we had a bit of explaining to do. Mam was a bit put out, as you'd expect, but at the end of the day everybody understood what drove us. I could die. I wanted Sarah to be my wife if I died. Nobody could argue with that.

CHAPTER THIRTEEN

'I'm a survivor'

We set about planning a family Christmas, and I allowed myself to slip into a brighter place than I had been since this ordeal had begun.

I wasn't in denial. I still faced more surgery, and I still felt tired and weak, but it was a relief to have no medical appointments to face until next year.

I started to talk to my agent about picking up work again, and when I was in London one afternoon I took myself off to Harvey Nichols and bought Sarah a fabulous pair of Christian Louboutin shoes for Christmas. It wasn't the first time I'd bought her designer shoes, but it felt like it. Just doing something as simple and normal as Christmas shopping felt like a gift. I was walking round London unaided, and it felt like a miracle. I enjoyed seeing the fairy lights strung along the street, and I looked up at their reflections in the thick city sky.

I'm not a religious man, or at least I am not a churchgoer. But I really felt my two mamgus, Annie and Lena, were looking down on me that day from heaven, twinkling happily in the sky and watching over me, like a couple of extra fairy lights.

Christmas Day itself was like so many other family Christmases that had gone before, and I was grateful for that. Mam and Dad came over, and so did Bec and Joni and my sister Victoria, her husband, Leigh, and little Livia. I got silly presents, like a Big Mouth Billy Bass singing fish, and my old man and I played a few games of darts.

I didn't eat the usual king-sized Christmas dinner I normally had, but I enjoyed every mouthful of what I did manage. Lina got a big pink tea set and made me pretend cups of tea, and I sat back and really relaxed. I'd forgotten what it was like to just enjoy spending time at home without thinking about drugs and hospitals.

By January I was well enough to commentate on a few matches, and the John Hartson Foundation was up and running, with new offices and a staff of six. I can't take the credit for that at all. Friends and family did most of the setting up for me. All I had to do was give it my unconditional backing and support, which was the easy bit.

Ryan Giggs and the rugby union stars Martin Johnson and Neil Jenkins came on board as patrons, and we started to organise our first fundraising events and build up a website. I wanted the main focus to be on raising awareness, so we decided to sell wristbands and give out posters, as well as getting me into schools and football clubs to give talks.

I was still going for regular blood tests to make sure my cancer markers stayed normal, which they did, but I worried less each time. My old life had come back to me, and I grabbed at it with both hands. I was driving my car, playing golf, seeing my friends and enjoying time with my kids.

Once or twice my body gave me a little reminder of what I'd been through. The first time was when I was watching Joni play football for the Swansea youth team one Sunday morning. One minute I was cheering him on, and the next I felt swamped with tiredness and had to ask one of the other parents to bring him home. I'd only been there for half an hour.

Another time I went to pick up a barrel of water from Mark's garage for our kitchen water cooler. He'd told me he'd carry it, but I tried to do it myself when he wasn't in. I got a few paces down the road and had to put it down. My lungs were struggling to pull in the air I needed. It made them sore just breathing, and my chest killed me for about four days afterwards. Sarah told me off and insisted I took things easier, but she was just weeks away from giving birth and I didn't think it was fair if I just collapsed on the sofa. Really, we both needed to rest more.

The midwife had advised Sarah to book in for an elective Caesarean this time round, given what had happened at Lina's birth. That was a huge relief to us both. Coping with another medical emergency was unthinkable.

The due date was 5 March, and this meant I could also plan the first operation on my lungs for the following week, 9 March, knowing Sarah would be home by then with the baby.

Ideally, the doctors would have liked to operate sooner, but I put them off. I didn't say it to Sarah, but the plain truth was I didn't want to die before my baby was born.

I'd been given a very detailed description of what the surgery entailed, and it was major. I felt slightly nauseous when the ins and outs were explained. Basically, the surgeon needed to cut the remaining 'lesions' or 'nodules' off my lungs so he could get them under a microscope and make sure they weren't cancerous. To do this, he needed to deflate each lung in turn in operations a month apart.

'We'll go into your back, cutting down about fourteen inches from the top of your shoulder blade . . . Then we'll open up the ribcage, use part of one of your ribs to clamp it open, deflate the left lung, feel around for any lesions, cut them off . . . Then we'll drill through the ribs and stitch you up from the inside. It should take about seven hours. We'll repeat the process on your right lung a month later, all being well.'

You can see why I felt a bit nauseous.

'You'll be fine, I'll be right here for you,' Sarah said breezily, and I said the same to her as we checked into the hospital for her Caesarean. My mother-in-law, Katherine, travelled with us to the Singleton for the birth. Our appointment was at 12.30 p.m.

'Have you decided on a name yet?' Katherine asked.

Sarah and I exchanged glances. This was one thing we hadn't managed to agree on.

'I like the name Belle,' Sarah said, going on to explain how she thought the baby looked like a 'wee bell' when we'd seen her on a special 4D scan we'd been asked to help promote.

'You're not calling her Belle,' I said. I just didn't like it. 'I like Florrie,' I said. 'I mean, your granny was Flora and there was Great Auntie Florrie . . .'

'You're not calling her Florrie,' Sarah said. 'I just don't like it enough.'

'What about Stephanie?' Katherine piped up from the back seat. 'I always imagine a Stephanie to be blonde . . .'

'I love that name!' I said, and we pulled into the Singleton Hospital car park.

This time it was my turn to support Sarah as she walked tentatively down the familiar corridors.

It was only a matter of months since I had been the patient here, but it suddenly felt like years. After Sarah's last antenatal appointment we'd been in to see my old nurses both here and at the Morriston, and I'd given them a hug and apologised for the moments when I'd given them a hard time. It had felt like peeping into the past. I barely remembered the rooms I had spent so many weeks in; they were just a distant memory. Now, with Sarah the one facing an operation, my own treatment was pushed even further back in my mind, and that's where I liked it.

I put on my blue scrubs and a brave smile, just as Sarah had done for me. I was delighted just to be here, and I couldn't quite believe that I was. 'I didn't think I would be around to see this,' I thought, remembering the dreadful fears I'd buried deep inside my head, frighteningly real fears of Sarah giving birth on her own.

'Good luck, babe,' I said. I was as nervous as hell. I held my breath, willing everything to go smoothly this time round. My heart rate quickened when I saw blood on Sarah's stomach, and then again when forceps were used to help pull our baby out into the world.

Then suddenly Stephanie was crying and screaming, and it was the best sound in the world. Her cry cut through absolutely everything. She had no hair and looked fabulous and pink as the midwife lifted her onto Sarah's chest. There was no emergency, no fear of losing her. It was a magical, perfect experience.

I nipped outside the delivery room to make a few phone calls and send a few texts. 'Stephanie Cari Hartson came into the world at 13.21 p.m. today . . . Mum and baby both fine . . . Fantastic news . . . 8 lb exactly . . .'

I posted it on Twitter later, too, and before I knew it the news of Stephanie's birth was in the *Evening Post* and the *Scottish Sun*.

'You're murder, John!' Sarah said, rolling her eyes.

We'd agreed on having Cari as the middle name, as it's Welsh for love, but I suddenly realised that picking the name Stephanie hadn't exactly been a unanimous and final decision.

'That's just typical of you, John. Slam, bam, job's done.' Thankfully Sarah laughed, albeit it in a rather world-weary way. She was too besotted with Stephanie to feel anything but delight.

When Lina met her new sister, it was a different story. She seemed to be fairly interested in Stephanie at first sight, but then threw herself face down on the floor wailing and screaming when she realised the baby was actually coming home with us that day – and was coming home to stay. Sarah and I looked at each other in mock horror. Life had just got busier, but we weren't complaining one bit.

We spent the next few days in a sort of baby blur, like you do. Stephanie demonstrated that she had a cracking pair of lungs on her, so much so that I barely had a moment to think about my own lungs and the two operations I faced.

When Stephanie was just four days old, Sarah and I beat the familiar route back to the Singleton for the first op, on my left lung. Stephanie slept soundly in her pram, oblivious to what was about to happen to her daddy. I kissed her on the forehead. 'I'll see you again very soon,' I told her.

'We'll be right here, waiting,' Sarah said. She gave me one of her brave, determined smiles. I'd got used to them by now. I knew she wouldn't give any head space to the inevitable fears she had. She never talked about 'what ifs', and I was grateful for that.

I knew I could die on the operating table. It was a major operation, and sometimes people just don't come back from something like that.

I also knew we could be in for more bad news. The shadows on my lungs – nodules, masses, lumps, tumours – call them what you like –

those things could still be concealing some cancerous cells that had hidden away, waiting to come back and get me.

Like Sarah, I kept those dark thoughts to myself, gritted my teeth and put my trust in the experts yet again.

'We took six nodules from your left lung,' I heard the doctor say. His voice sounded muffled. I was waking up, and I was alive. 'It has all gone according to plan.'

I felt sick and drowsy, and I had an uncomfortable pain running all the way down the left-hand side of my back, but I was alive.

'Look at the state of us, what a pair!' I remember Sarah smiling the next day, when I was discharged. Stephanie was asleep in her car seat. It felt like I had only missed minutes of her life, not a whole day.

'Let's go, what are we waiting for?' I asked Sarah. I felt groggy and exhausted, but I was dressed, my bag was packed and I wanted to get home as quickly as possible.

We both looked at Stephanie, sleeping soundly in her car seat, and the penny dropped. Sarah had arrived at the hospital at the same time as a friend, who had carried Stephanie from the car. Now we had no help, and one of us had to carry Stephanie back to the car in her bulky car seat and drive home. We didn't want to disturb the baby, but suddenly she seemed like an impossibly heavy package, buckled in her well-padded carrier. We had no pram, as we'd had the day before when I had driven us to the hospital, and now I wasn't even allowed to drive, let alone carry Stephanie.

'I can't lift her in that seat,' we both said at the same time. We dissolved into laughter, Sarah clutching her five-day-old Caesarean scar, me wincing in pain and feeling like my back had been attacked by a samurai sword instead of a surgeon's delicate knife.

Somehow we hauled a still-sleeping Stephanie out to the car between us, and Sarah got in the driving seat. 'You're not supposed to drive for six weeks,' I told her.

'Well, how do you think I got home yesterday? I'm more likely to do myself an injury loading the washing machine than driving an automatic Volvo, now get in,' she told me.

I entered a two-week wait for the results from my lung op, and it was a long and nervous wait, I don't mind admitting. I tried to fill my days as best I could, but with the massive scar I found it hard to sleep, and I was tired and restless.

I couldn't possibly swing a golf club, so the driving range was out. I could think about the Foundation, though, and one morning I came up with a great idea.

'Why don't we do a charity walk up Ben Nevis on 14 July?' I said to Sarah. 'We could raise loads of money, and it would mark the anniversary of the day I stopped breathing. I said I'd do the climb anyway when I was better, and I might as well turn it into a fundraising opportunity.'

'Great idea, I'll do it with you,' Sarah said, just like that.

I also fixed up lots of TV work, mainly for the local Welsh-speaking channel S4C, and I agreed to appear as a guest on *Soccer AM* and ESPN's *Talk of the Terrace*.

I was feeling less like a cancer patient and more like a survivor, and when the lung mass results finally came back from the lab as 'inactive', I was relieved but not particularly surprised by them. Normality was gradually returning.

'I'd have been surprised if they hadn't come back normal,' Sarah said, and I had to agree.

I phoned everyone with the news. 'My left lung is all clear!' I said triumphantly. I could feel my anxiety dissolving.

'Is that it then, John, are you cancer-free?' friends and colleagues asked.

I had to explain that I was to return to hospital in four weeks to undergo the exact same process on my right lung. 'There's no reason why the right shouldn't be the same as the left,' I said confidently. 'They don't expect to find any live cancer cells there either.'

To be truthful, I don't think the doctors had made such cavalier predictions; they were usually more cautious than that. Nevertheless, as I waited for the second lung op I believed my own publicity wholeheartedly. I was sure this was a formality now, even though there was still a quiet little voice lurking in the back of my head that hissed dark thoughts sometimes, usually when I couldn't sleep in the early hours of the morning. 'You could die, you know, John. Your luck could run out, Big Man.' It said things like that, but I tried not to listen. I didn't really think it was true any more.

A couple of weeks before my next surgery, I was invited to Downing Street. Sarah Brown was hosting a 'Beating Cancer in This Generation' function, and I readily agreed to attend. It was an honour just to walk in through the famous front door of Number 10 and up the staircase with all the ex-prime ministers' portraits looking down on me.

'There's not many lads from my block who've done this,' I thought to myself.

I was shown into a crowded room, and Sarah Brown came over for a chat. She said 'well done' to me for winning my personal battle with cancer, and also for helping raise awareness.

I then stood at the back of the crowd and waited for the Health Secretary, Andy Burnham, to give a talk about beating cancer.

I spotted Denise van Outen and Nicola from Girls Aloud, and was enjoying being part of such a high-profile event, when all of a sudden Andy Burnham singled me out and spoke about my cancer battle for a good couple of minutes. The whole room clapped, and I felt myself going bright red, but I felt ten feet tall, too. It gave me a real boost, and I knew then that the Foundation was exactly the right thing for me to pour my energy into.

When you're a cancer patient, I think you sometimes look for signs and explanations. You inevitably think 'why me?', but if you're lucky you can see beyond the unfairness of it all. The meeting at Downing Street made me focus firmly on the positive. I was in a position to raise awareness, and maybe that was the answer to that inevitable question: 'Why me?'

I held onto this thought as the days edged towards my second lung operation.

'It'll be fine,' I told Sarah. 'It'll be a carbon copy of the last op. It'll look like I've been attacked by two samurai swords, not one. I'll have matching scars and matching results.'

Thankfully, I turned out to be right. Two weeks on, the lab results came back negative once again. There was just one large nodule on my right lung, and it was completely cancer-free. Despite my optimism, I can't say I wasn't mightily relieved.

'I knew it would be clear,' Sarah said. 'Only one more hurdle to jump now, John. I told you you'd be right as rain in time for the wedding party.'

It was springtime now, and I felt myself getting stronger almost by the day.

The next step was to have another brain scan, to see if I needed to have any further surgery to mop up any nodules left in my head. After that I'd be home and dry; that's what I told myself.

When the date came through for the brain appointment – 2 June – I decided to write it in my diary. Work with the Foundation was building up. We had lots of events planned, my TV jobs were increasing and I was being asked to help promote blood donations and give talks in schools and at football clubs.

I didn't want to turn anyone down. I'd learned I'd had two blood transfusions in hospital during my treatment, so I would have died if others hadn't donated blood. I'd had phenomenal support from young football fans, some of whom were affected by cancer too. I wanted to give as much back as I possibly could. I enjoyed becoming a busy man again, but I realised I needed to get more organised.

I couldn't find my diary at first. Usually I left it in my car, but I rooted through the glove compartment and it wasn't there. I eventually found it under a pile of papers in the office, and I opened it with the thin red ribbon that acts as a bookmark.

It fell open on Thursday, 9 July 2009 – the last time I'd used it – and there were two entries sitting innocently side by side: 'Scan, Neath Port Talbot Hospital, 3.25 p.m.' and 'S4C commentary box, Llanelli v. Motherwell, 6 p.m.'.

I stared at the page. It was the first time I had remembered that day in any detail. How could I have been so naïve as to think I could commentate on a UEFA match when I had felt so ill? How did I not realise the significance of my headaches, when I had lumps on my testicle that were getting bigger, not smaller? How could I have not even considered that the scan might tell me I had testicular cancer?

I exhaled slowly. Looking back, seeing that scan appointment in black and white, it all seemed so clear, so obvious. But when I was living through it, I couldn't see a thing. I didn't want to see what was happening to me. I thought I could barge my way through life, and until that point, that's exactly what I did.

I started flicking through the pages. July, August, September: they were all blank. I turned them quickly, because it felt so uncomfortable seeing so many empty pages. My life had stopped. October, November, December: there was nothing there at all.

I grabbed a pen and started scribbling in every date I could remember off the top of my head, turning the pages to fill the white spaces with Stephanie's birthday (5 March), our wedding day (4 December) and going forward to add the Ben Nevis climb (14 July), a world record 50-hour football match attempt I was kicking off (7 May), and our big wedding party (23 July).

Finally I wrote 'brain scan' on 2 June, and I suddenly remembered I was getting my teeth whitened the following week, so I jotted down my dental appointment too.

I felt so relieved to have my life back in my own hands, and for a brain scan to be slotted into my diary just like a trip to the dentist.

Underneath my diary I found Victoria's diary, written in black ink in a ring binder patterned with brightly coloured spots. She had handed it to me when I left hospital, and I had started to read it, but I became too emotional. Just reading about all my visitors and the support I received had made me cry, and I didn't feel strong enough to read all about my treatment and how close I came to death's door.

Now, though, I felt the urge to fill in that void left in my own diary.

I quietly shut the office door and read every word my little sister had written. I cried, but when I turned the last page I felt strangely elated, too.

Tuesday, 29 September 2009

John,

I hope you've had a good insight reading this description of what you've been going through since 10 July. Your family will always remain by your side, and you've got such a lovely future to look forward to with Sarah, Lina and the new baby due in March.

We're all very proud of you. Joni and Bec idolise you, and you've put up such a great fight so far.

Bring it on!

All my love for ever, Vic xx

I had survived. I was filling in my own diary again. The new baby was here. Life was going on, just as it should. I phoned Vic and thanked her for what she had done, and I told her she had done a great thing and, with her permission, I was going to publish the diary to help raise awareness.

'My cancer story would have ended almost before it began had I faced the lump four or five years earlier than I did,' I told her.

'Everything that happened to me, everything I put my family and friends through, could have been avoided if I'd faced the lump sooner.

'I want people to know I very nearly died, and it could happen to them if they ignore the warning signs. Thank you so much for everything you've done.'

'John, you're my hero,' Vic said. 'It's your life and your story. I just wrote it down. The rest is up to you.'

In May, freelance work rolled in thick and fast. I still had my weekly *Sun* column, but the S4C work meant that for the first time in over a year Sarah and I could feel completely comfortable about our finances again.

I remembered my producer, Emyr's, words when I told him I had just been diagnosed with testicular cancer. He was the first person I had told. 'I'm devastated for you,' he had said. 'Go and get yourself well, John. Get yourself fit and we'll see you back.' I couldn't believe I was going back so soon, and it seemed very fitting to be returning to S4C.

A couple of months earlier I'd been offered a three-year deal to manage Barry Town, and I'd reluctantly turned it down. I felt the timing wasn't quite right, what with the new baby arriving and me still having operations. I also felt very loyal to the media companies that had stuck by me during my illness, so I was delighted to have a steady

TV job again. Besides, it would keep me in the public eye and help me raise awareness.

On 2 June I went in for my brain scan and a consultation, as planned. My lungs were clear, and I felt sure my brain would be too. My meetings with Dr Bertelli were fewer and further between now, and they were less fraught each time. This one didn't really bother me. I was sure my brain was clear. If I'd had live cancer cells I'd have been shocked, but, of course, the possibility was still there.

Dr Bertelli's encouraging smile spoke volumes to me again before he opened his mouth. 'There is a large tumour at the back of your head, but it is dead,' he told me. 'There is no cancerous activity going on. It is just sitting there.'

He went on to say that we had three options. Number one: they could open up my skull and attempt to clear it away, just as they had scraped the nodules off my lungs. Number two: try to blast it away with a laser. Number three: absolutely nothing.

I had been through so many operations in just nine months, from the emergency brain surgery to having the drain internalised, and the tracheotomy, and finally the two lung operations. Undergoing another general anaesthetic was to be avoided if at all possible, so for the time being we agreed to do nothing at all.

I walked out of the hospital feeling buoyant with relief. It wasn't quite over yet. I still had a dead tumour in my head, which wasn't exactly great, but my body was now officially cancer-free. My decline had been incredibly rapid, but so too had my recovery. I would have to have scans and blood tests every few months, and my results would have to be negative for five years before I was given the official all-clear, but I was technically in remission. My treatment had been overwhelmingly successful.

'The only way is up,' I joked to Sarah that night. She was organising our transport and walking gear for the Ben Nevis climb, now just a few weeks' away. She'd conquered the mountain several times before and was full of confidence, but she knew I was nervous.

'I've said it before and I'll say it again, I've never doubted you, John,' Sarah said. 'I was 100 per cent certain the chemo had worked on your brain tumour, and I know you'll have no trouble reaching the top of Ben Nevis. You'll eat it for breakfast.'

I really hoped she was right. I'd started bulking up my muscles with a tough fitness routine over the past few weeks. I boxed in the gym like a madman, and I took part in the Llanelli Waterside 10 k, just to see if I could do it. I did complete it, even though I must admit I had to walk and jog slowly most of the way and my lungs hurt like mad.

My parents were concerned that I was overdoing things, but I told them, 'I need to look and feel more like my old self, more like "Big Bad John" if I am going to conquer that monster of a mountain.' By the time 14 July came around, my weight had increased to 16 st. and I had familiar bulging muscles in my legs and arms again. I was delighted, and I was ready for the challenge. It felt like such a big day, and I was determined to succeed. It was Lina's birthday, exactly two years to the day when she had arrived in the world not breathing, and it was exactly one year to the day when I had stopped breathing in hospital. Now it was going to also be the day Sarah and I climbed a mountain together. Another one.

The weather was atrocious. Wind and rain battered my face as I looked towards the summit. It was hidden behind a screen of mist some 4,406 ft away from me and it felt impossibly far away, but I gritted my teeth and put one foot in front of the other over and over again, for more than four hours.

I can honestly say it was the hardest thing I have ever done in my life. My lungs ached, my legs buckled and each step I took seemed to be steeper and tougher than the one before. It was worse than enduring chemo, worse than pre-season training and worse than tackling any of the toughest footballers in the world. In hospital and on the pitch I had incredible teams behind me, but now it was all down to me. It was my personal battle, and only I could take each and every step forward.

When the summit finally came into view after four hours and fifteen minutes, the tears came pouring out. I just couldn't stop them. More than 60 other climbers had made the ascent with me, helping to raise thousands of pounds for cancer charities and the hospitals that had treated me so well. Most had beaten me to the finish, and many were concerned I wouldn't make it. When I finally appeared, smiling in the face of 65 mph gusts of wind, they started to chant, 'There's only one Johnny Hartson . . . he's got no hair but we don't care . . . walking in a Hartson wonderland.'

I flung my arms around Sarah and sobbed. I was completely overwhelmed. I gasped for breath, but I couldn't be sure if I was breathless with the effort of the climb or breathless at what I had achieved. I waved a victory flag above my head, filled my tired lungs with fresh mountain air and felt amazingly alive. I had the world at my feet, just like my dad had always told me. 'I did it,' I said, hugging Sarah. 'I'm a survivor – and I couldn't have made this journey without you.'

John's epilogue

I tackled cancer in the same way I played professional football. I called on all my physical strength, gritted my teeth and got stuck in with all my might. You can't shy away or tremble on the sidelines or you lose, just like you do in football. If you want to beat cancer, you have to put up the biggest fight of your life. Do I think you have to be a strong and positive person to beat cancer? Not necessarily. I might have looked indestructible on the football pitch, but throughout my life I've had moments of self-doubt and times when I've felt the world was crashing in, just like anybody else. There were low points in my treatment when the pain was so bad I thought, 'I can't make it through.' I don't think positive thinking alone can get you through those black times. I believe in God. I think there must be something up there, and I'm not frightened. Being a dad is ultimately what kept me fighting. Thinking I would never see my children again gave me the strength to battle on. When you are faced with that terrible thought you fight like hell for your life, whether you're a big, tough footballer or not. I don't want to miss out on watching my kids grow up, and I am going to look after myself so much better from now on. I am convinced the lack of respect I had for my body and the stress I caused myself in my personal life played a part in my cancer, but, of course, I will never know for sure. I want to be a better person for Sarah's sake, both in terms of looking after myself and sorting out my gambling habit once and for all. She deserves the best I can give her. Cancer has shown me what a very special person she is. She has supported me tirelessly, and we are closer than ever. I want to say thank you to all my amazing family and friends who showed me so much support.

Hopefully my story will improve or even save the lives of others. I don't want anybody else to suffer because of their ignorance.

Sarah's epilogue

John used to live life at full blast, like he was running through every day on a treadmill, and I was happy to keep up the pace. Cancer stopped us in our tracks. It's only now, a year on, that I can really reflect. It took a long time for the events of last summer to sink in. John got ill really quickly, then almost as quickly he started to get better. When things were bad I couldn't let myself get too melancholy. I couldn't go to that freaky place where he nearly died. It's only now that we've got through it and been able to take our breath that I can think, 'I nearly lost him.' Now we focus more on the here and now. We appreciate what and who is important in our lives, and we try not to let little things bother us any more. I am learning to stop and think if I feel irritated or annoyed. I ask myself: 'Is it important? Does it really matter?' Usually the answer is no. The trick I have learned from all this is to try your best to live each day as if it's your last, and don't take anything for granted. John and I felt as giddy and excited as a couple of teenagers when we sat down together to plan our wedding party. Perhaps before cancer we would have moaned about the never-ending arrangements instead of enjoying perfecting each and every detail to make our big day special. Now, every day with John is big and special.

Blitz

rosebay willowherb.

98% loss of flora meadow

Thale cress -
   genetic stats because of speed
of reproduction

cress - quech - die -
   humus - often follow -
bramble - break up ground
oxygen - clover - nitogen -
bracken - humus - substrata -
moss - saplings -
         ↓
beech, oak -